About the NCCN Guidelines for Patients®

National Comprehensive Cancer Network®

AF884857

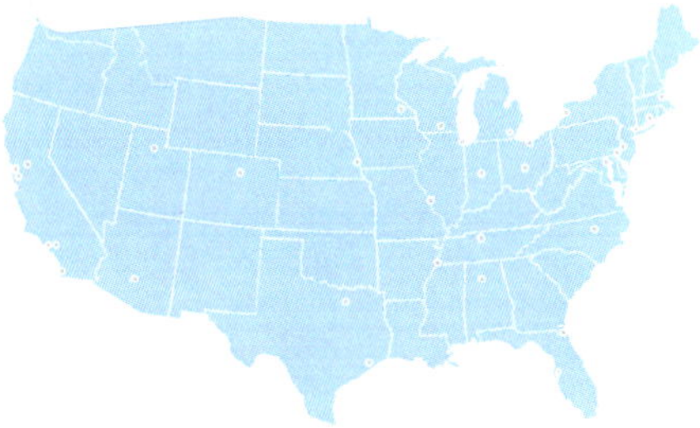

Did you know that top cancer centers across the United States work together to improve cancer care? This alliance of leading cancer centers is called the National Comprehensive Cancer Network® (NCCN®).

Cancer care is always changing. NCCN develops evidence-based cancer care recommendations used by health care providers worldwide. These frequently updated recommendations are the NCCN Clinical Practice Guidelines in Oncology (NCCN Guidelines®). The NCCN Guidelines for Patients plainly explain these expert recommendations for people with cancer and caregivers.

These NCCN Guidelines for Patients are based on the NCCN Clinical Practice Guidelines in Oncology (NCCN Guidelines®) for Cervical Cancer, Version 4.2025 — March 24, 2025.

Learn how the NCCN Guidelines for Patients are developed
NCCN.org/patient-guidelines-process

View the NCCN Guidelines for Patients free online
NCCN.org/patientguidelines

Find an NCCN Cancer Center near you
NCCN.org/cancercenters

Connect with us YouTube

Supporters

NCCN Guidelines for Patients are supported by funding from the NCCN Foundation®

NCCN Foundation gratefully acknowledges the following corporate supporters for helping to make available these NCCN Guidelines for Patients: Pfizer Inc.

NCCN independently adapts, updates, and hosts the NCCN Guidelines for Patients. Our corporate supporters do not participate in the development of the NCCN Guidelines for Patients and are not responsible for the content and recommendations contained therein.

Additional support is provided by

Ovarian Cancer Research Alliance is committed to curing ovarian cancer, advocating for patients, and supporting survivors. OCRA is the largest ovarian cancer charity with over $128 million invested in research. Our national conference, webinars, and website offer the most up to date information on diagnosis, treatment and living with ovarian and gynecologic cancers. Our programs include our Patient Support line, peer mentor program, Staying Connected support series, 1:1 Counseling, Clinical Trial Navigator, and genetic testing program. OCRA builds community through advocacy, research, collaboration, and support. For more information, please visit ocrahope.org or call 212-268-1002.

To make a gift or learn more, visit online or email

NCCNFoundation.org/donate

PatientGuidelines@NCCN.org

Contents

NCCN Foundation seeks to support the millions of patients and their families affected by a cancer diagnosis by funding and distributing NCCN Guidelines for Patients. NCCN Foundation is also committed to advancing cancer treatment by funding the nation's promising doctors at the center of innovation in cancer research. For more details and the full library of patient and caregiver resources, visit NCCN.org/patients.

National Comprehensive Cancer Network (NCCN) and NCCN Foundation
3025 Chemical Road, Suite 100, Plymouth Meeting, PA 19462 USA

1
About cervical cancer

Most cervical cancers are caused by long-term infection with human papillomavirus (HPV), a common sexually transmitted infection. The most common type is squamous cell carcinoma (SCC).

The cervix

The uterus is where a baby grows and develops during pregnancy. The cervix is the narrow, lower end of the uterus. During birth, the cervix opens and thins to allow the baby to move into the vagina.

The ectocervix is the outer, rounded part of the cervix that extends into the vagina. In the center is a narrow opening called the external os. During your period, the external os opens slightly to allow blood to pass into the vagina.

The endocervix is the inner part of the cervix that forms a canal between the vagina and the body of the uterus. The inner os is the upper part of the endocervix that serves as an opening between the uterus and the cervix.

The area where the endocervix and ectocervix meet is called the squamocolumnar junction or the transformation zone. Most cervical cancers and pre-cancers start in the ectocervix portion of the transformation zone.

Uterine cancer is diagnosed and treated differently than cervical cancer. This patient guide doesn't discuss treatment of uterine

The cervix

Most cervical cancers start in the area where the inner and outer cervix meet, called the squamocolumnar junction. Specifically, most form in squamous cells that line the ectocervix part of the squamocolumnar junction.

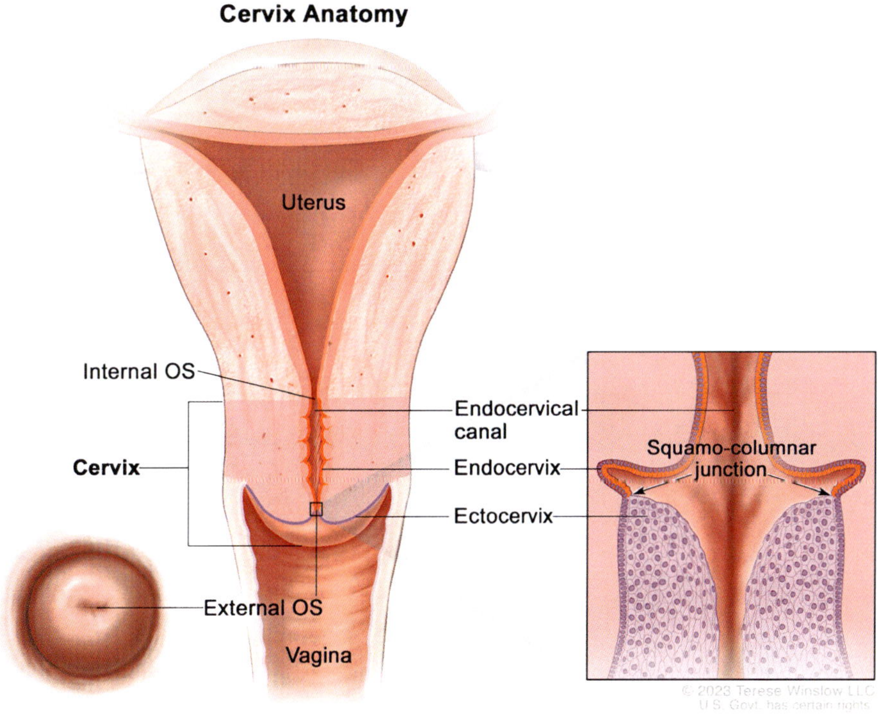

cancers, such as endometrial cancer and uterine sarcomas.

How does cervical cancer start?

Cervical cancer starts as lesions (areas) of abnormal cells on the surface of the cervix. These microscopic changes are known as cervical dysplasia or cervical intraepithelial neoplasia (CIN). If left untreated, cervical dysplasia may become cervical cancer.

CIN is graded based on how deep the abnormal cells extend into the lining of the cervix. The possible grades are 1, 2, or 3. Cervical dysplasia becomes cancer when the abnormal cells invade the muscular tissue beneath the cervical lining (the cervical stroma).

Low-grade squamous intraepithelial lesion (LSIL) refers to mild dysplasia (CIN 1). High-grade squamous intraepithelial lesion (HSIL) refers to moderate or severe dysplasia (CIN 2 and 3), and is considered a pre-cancer.

Cervical changes

Cervical dysplasia refers to areas of abnormal cells on the lining of the cervix. LSIL refers to mild dysplasia (CIN 1). HSIL refers to moderate or severe dysplasia (CIN 2 and 3), and is considered a pre-cancer.

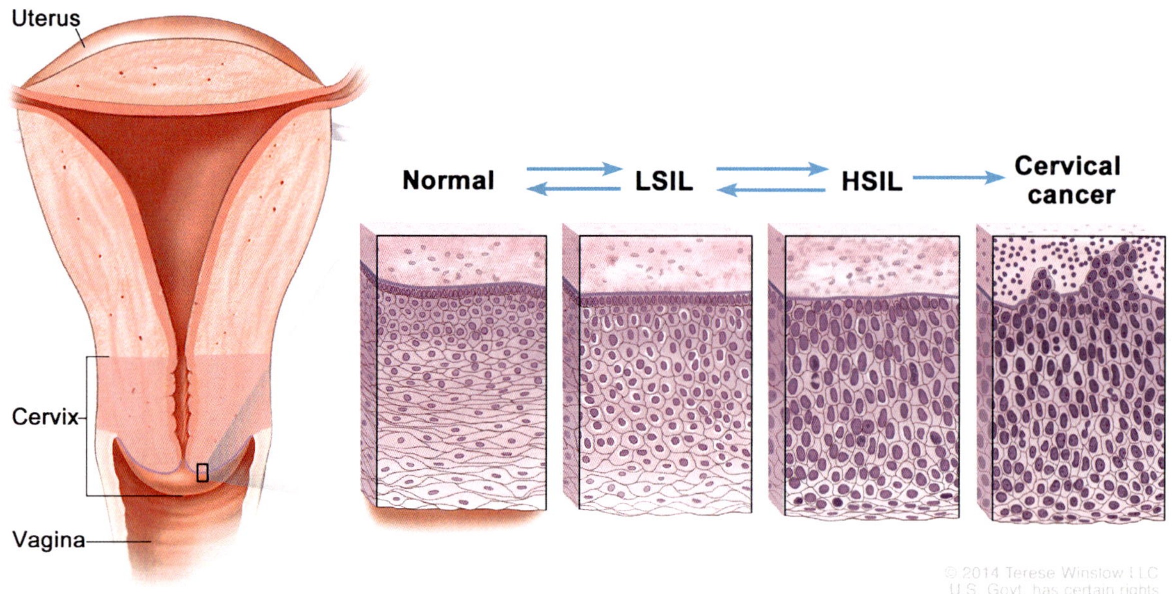

Who is most at risk?

A risk factor is something that increases the risk of developing a disease. Some people with no known risk factors may develop cervical cancer, while others with risk factors may not.

HPV infection

Almost all cervical cancers are caused by long-term infection with human papillomavirus (HPV). HPV is a common sexually transmitted infection (STI). Most sexually active people have or had HPV at some point. Most are unaware that they are or were infected.

In most people, the immune system gets rid of HPV from the body. In other people, the virus causes long-term cell changes that develop into cancer, often decades after the initial infection. Experts are still learning why one person gets cervical cancer and another does not. Other types of cancer caused by HPV include anal, head and neck, penile, vaginal, and vulvar cancers.

There are more than 100 types (strains) of HPV. Infection with some strains is more likely to lead to cancer. High-risk forms include HPV-16 and HPV-18. Other HPV types can cause abnormal skin growths, called warts, to form on the anus, genitals, or other areas of the body.

A vaccine that protects against 9 different strains of HPV, including the highest-risk strains, is available in the United States.

Before, vaccination was only recommended for routine use in adolescents and young adults. Now it is an option for adults aged 45 and under. There are 2 other HPV vaccines available in other parts of the world. One protects against HPV-16 and HPV-18 only. The other targets these and 2 more types.

The vaccine works best in younger people (ideally under age 13) because they are less likely to have been exposed to HPV. And, while the vaccine can prevent new HPV infections, it doesn't treat existing HPV infections or HPV-related cancer.

Other risk factors

Other risk factors for cervical cancer are listed below. Some of these lead to a higher risk because they either increase the risk of being exposed to HPV or they weaken the immune system, which can make it harder for the body to clear HPV infection.

- A history of smoking
- Having given birth more than once (called high parity or multiparity)
- Oral contraceptive (birth control) use
- Being sexually active at an early age
- A high number of sexual partners
- A history of sexually transmitted infection
- Certain autoimmune diseases
- A weakened immune system due to HIV or AIDS, for example

Types of cervical cancer

Most cervical cancers start in the ectocervix, which is lined with squamous cells. Cancers that form here are called squamous cell carcinomas.

About 1 in 5 cervical cancers form in the endocervix, which is lined with glandular cells that make mucus. Cancers that form in glandular cells are called adenocarcinomas.

Less commonly, the cancer may contain both squamous and adenocarcinoma cells. These are referred to as adenosquamous carcinomas or "mixed" tumors. The rarest and most aggressive type of cervical cancer is neuroendocrine carcinoma of the cervix (NECC).

This patient guide doesn't discuss other types of cervical cancer such as glassy cell carcinomas, sarcomas, or other tumor types.

Why you should read this book

Making decisions about cancer care can be stressful. You may need to make tough decisions under pressure about complex choices.

The NCCN Guidelines for Patients are trusted by patients and providers. They clearly explain current care recommendations made by respected experts in the field. Recommendations are based on the latest research and practices at leading cancer centers.

Cancer care is not the same for everyone. By following expert recommendations for your situation, you are more likely to improve your care and have better outcomes as a result. Use this book as your guide to find the information you need to make important decisions.

What can you do to get the best care?

Advocate for yourself. You're more likely to get the care you want by asking questions and making shared decisions with your care team.

The NCCN Guidelines for Patients will help you understand cancer care. With better understanding, you'll be more prepared to discuss your care with your team and share your concerns. Many people feel more satisfied when they play an active role in their care.

You may not know what to ask your care team. That's common. Each chapter in this book ends with an important section called *Questions to ask.* These suggested questions will help you get more information on all aspects of your care.

2
Testing for cervical cancer

Your provider will make a treatment plan just for you. First, they will gather information about the cancer and your general health. This chapter describes testing and other care needed to create your treatment plan.

Cervical biopsy

A cervical biopsy involves removing small samples of tissue from the cervix. It's the most commonly used procedure to diagnose cervical cancer. Samples may be taken from the ectocervix, the endocervix, or both.

The removed tissue is examined by a pathologist. A pathologist is a doctor who specializes in evaluating cells and tissues to diagnose disease. They look for abnormal areas, including areas of cancer or pre-cancer. The pathologist also determines the type of cervical cancer, when possible.

Cervical biopsy

A cervical biopsy is the most commonly used procedure to diagnose cervical cancer. A small sample of tissue is removed from the ectocervix, the endocervix, or both.

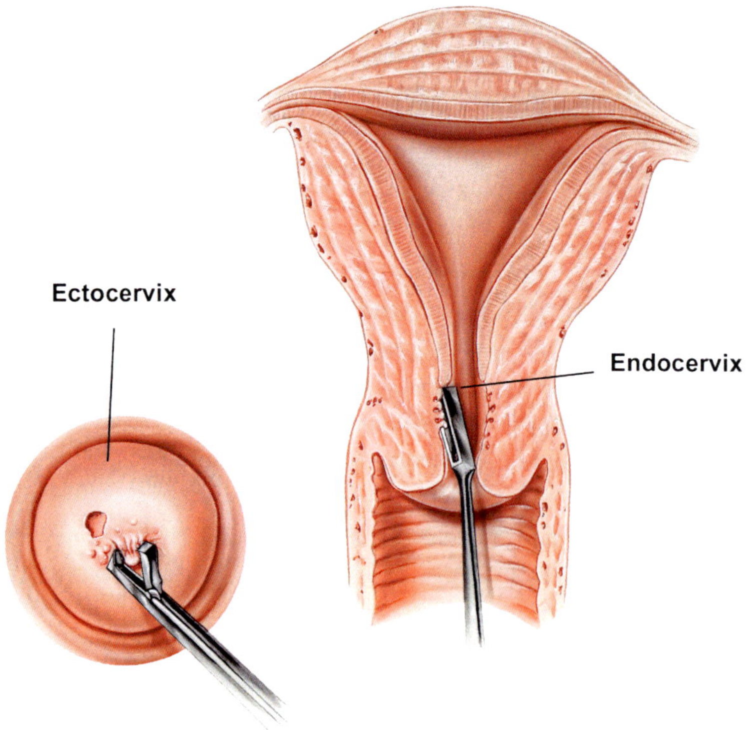

Cone biopsy

Cone biopsy can be both a test and a treatment. It involves removing a cone-shaped portion of the cervix.

The cone-shaped sample includes tissue from both the ectocervix and the endocervical canal. All of the transformation zone—where the ectocervix and endocervix meet—is removed. Most cervical cancers start in this area.

Most commonly, a technique called cold knife conization is used. In this method a surgical scalpel is used to remove the tissue. In some cases loop electrosurgical excision procedure (LEEP) may be performed instead. In LEEP, a thin loop of electrified (heated) wire is used instead of a scalpel to cut out the cervical tissue.

After removing the cone-shaped sample of tissue, your doctor may use a spoon-like tool called a curette to scrape a sample of tissue from the cervical canal. This is called endocervical curettage.

The tissue removed during a cone biopsy is examined under a microscope by a pathologist.

Cone biopsy

A cone biopsy removes a cone-shaped section of the cervix that includes the transformation zone. Cone biopsy may be the only treatment needed for some early-stage cervical cancers.

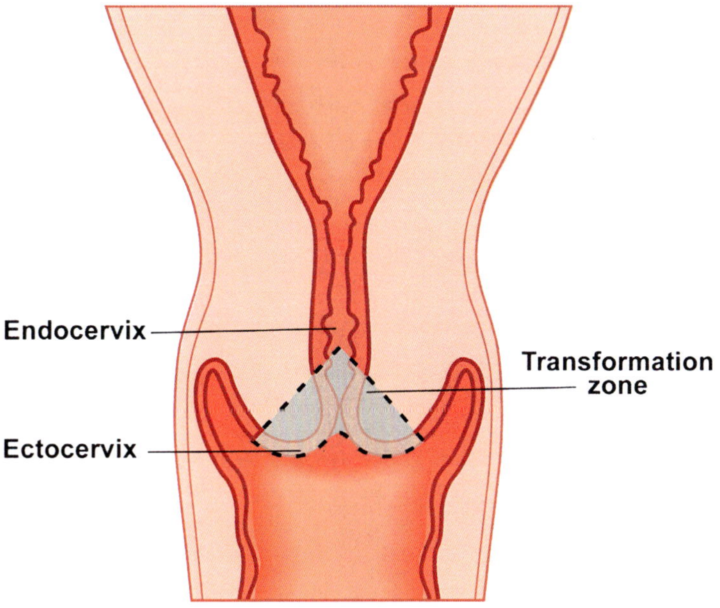

Blood tests

The following blood tests may be ordered as part of initial testing. They provide helpful information about your general health and the health of your liver, kidneys, and other organs before treatment.

A complete blood count (CBC) is a common test that measures the number of red blood cells, white blood cells, and platelets in a sample of blood. Red blood cells carry oxygen throughout the body. White blood cells fight infection. Platelets help to control bleeding.

A blood chemistry profile measures the levels of different chemicals in your blood. Chemicals in your blood are affected by your kidneys, bones, and other organs and tissues. Blood chemistry levels that are too high or too low may be a sign that an organ is not working well. Abnormal levels may also be caused by the spread of cancer or by other diseases.

Liver function tests are often done along with a blood chemistry profile. The liver is an organ that does many important jobs, such as remove toxins from the blood. Liver function tests measure enzymes that are made or processed by the liver. Levels that are too high or too low may be a sign of liver damage or cancer spread.

If you haven't had a recent human immunodeficiency virus (HIV) test, or have never been tested, your provider may recommend it. If you have HIV, you are likely to be referred to an HIV specialist. Having HIV should not affect your cancer treatment. The treatment options described in this guide apply to patients who are HIV-positive or HIV-negative.

Imaging

Imaging helps determine the extent of the cancer. The size and spread of the cancer is used to guide treatment.

Computed tomography

You may have a computed tomography (CT) scan of your chest, abdomen, and pelvis. A CT scan is a more detailed kind of x-ray. It takes many pictures of an area inside the body from different angles. A computer combines the pictures to make three-dimensional (3D) images.

During the scan, you will lie face up on a table that moves through a large tunnel-like machine. To see everything better, a substance called contrast may be injected into your vein and also mixed with a liquid you drink. Contrast makes the CT pictures clearer.

The contrast may cause you to feel flushed or get hives. You will be able to hear and talk to the technician at all times. You may hear buzzing or clicking during the scan.

PET/CT

CT may be combined with positron emission tomography (PET). PET uses small amounts of radioactive materials called radiotracers. About an hour before the scan, you will be injected with a sugar radiotracer. The radiotracer gives off a small amount of energy that can be seen by the imaging machine. Cancer appears brighter in the pictures because cancer cells use sugar more quickly than normal cells.

In some cases, PET may be performed with magnetic resonance imaging (MRI) (described next) instead of CT.

Magnetic resonance imaging

You may have an MRI of your pelvis. MRI uses magnetic fields and radio waves to make detailed pictures of the uterus, cervix, and vagina. An MRI may show whether the cancer has spread to tissues next to the cervix, such as the parametrium, vagina, bladder, or rectum.

For those with small cell neuroendocrine carcinoma of the cervix (NECC), MRI of the brain is also recommended as part of initial testing.

Getting an MRI scan is similar to getting a CT scan, but takes longer. You will lie face-up on a table that moves through a large tunnel in the scanning machine. The scan may cause your body to feel a bit warm. A contrast agent will be used to make the pictures clearer. Tell your provider if you get nervous in tight spaces.

Transvaginal ultrasound

If you cannot have MRI of your pelvis, you may have an ultrasound instead. Ultrasound uses sound waves to make pictures of areas inside of the body. It is good at showing the size, shape, and location of the cervix.

In a transvaginal ultrasound, a probe will be inserted into your vagina. This helps your doctor see the cervix and nearby areas more clearly.

MRI

An MRI makes pictures of areas inside the body without using radiation. An MRI can show the tissues of the uterus, cervix, and vagina in detail.

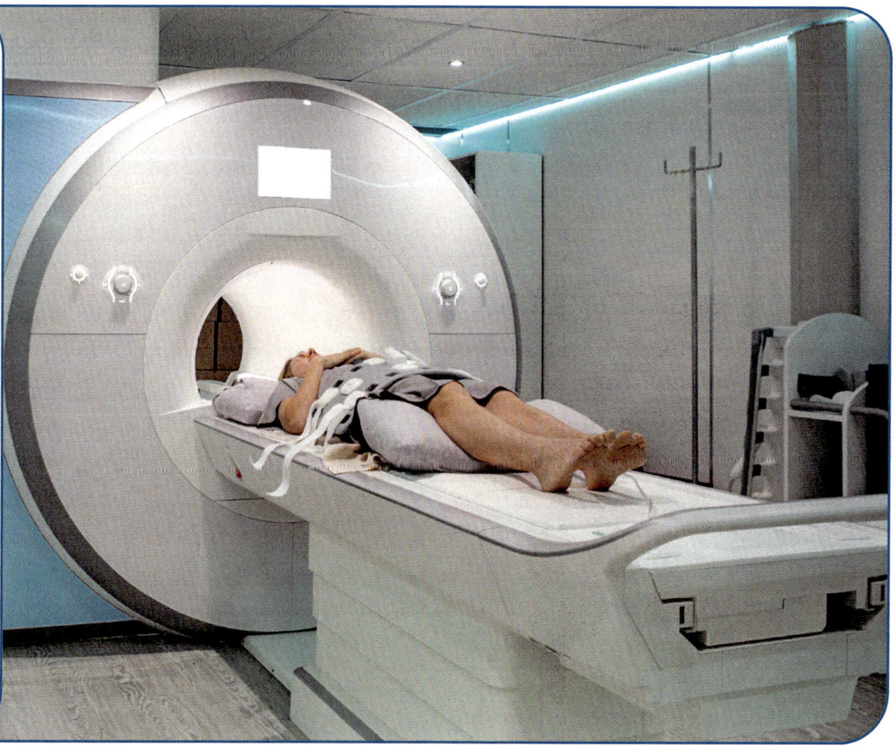

Fertility and pregnancy

If you want the option of becoming pregnant in the future, talk to your care team about fertility-sparing treatment. It is typically only an option for small, early-stage cancers. Recommendations for fertility-sparing treatment are provided in *Chapter 5: Treatment for common types*.

If fertility preservation is desired, talk to your provider about seeing a reproductive endocrinologist. Reproductive endocrinologists are doctors that specialize in fertility. Although natural pregnancy will not be possible in most cases, options to discuss may include ovarian transposition, egg or embryo freezing, and consideration of possible surrogate pregnancy in the future.

Ovarian transposition

Cervical cancer treatment may involve external beam radiation therapy (EBRT). Radiation damages the ovaries and causes them to stop producing hormones needed for natural pregnancy. Ovarian transposition is a surgery that moves one or both ovaries out of the range of the radiation beam. The medical name for this procedure is oophoropexy.

Ovarian transposition before starting EBRT may be an option if you are premenopausal and have the most common type of cervical cancer, squamous cell carcinoma.

Egg freezing

Unfertilized eggs can be removed, frozen, and stored for later use. Another name for this is oocyte preservation.

Surrogacy

If you have frozen embryos or frozen eggs (oocytes), you may consider using a surrogate. A surrogate (often a relative or friend) volunteers to have the embryos inserted into their uterus. They carry the pregnancy and give birth.

For more information on fertility preservation, see the *NCCN Guidelines for Patients: Adolescent and Young Adult Cancer* at NCCN.org/patientguidelines and on the NCCN Patient Guides for Cancer app.

Bladder and bowel tests

Your provider may want to examine nearby organs, like the bladder and bowel, for signs of cancer. If these tests are needed, expect to receive general anesthesia. This means you will be fully sedated and unaware that the procedure is taking place. These are referred to as examinations under anesthesia (EUAs).

Cystoscopy is a procedure to see inside the bladder and other organs of the urinary tract. It is performed using a hollow tool with a magnifying lens at one end, called a cystoscope. The cystoscope is inserted through the urethra and guided into the bladder.

Proctoscopy is a procedure to see inside the anus and rectum. It is performed with a thin, tube-like instrument with a light and magnifying lens called a proctoscope.

If abnormal or suspicious areas are seen during cystoscopy or proctoscopy, tissue samples will be removed and tested (biopsied).

Cancer care plan

Your care team

Treatment for cervical cancer often involves a team of experts, including a gynecologic oncologist, a medical oncologist, and a radiation oncologist.

A gynecologic oncologist is an expert in surgery and chemotherapy for female reproductive cancers. A medical oncologist is an expert in treating cancer with systemic therapies (medicines), like chemotherapy. A radiation oncologist is an expert in the use of radiation therapy to treat cancer.

Other health care providers that you see for routine care can also be a part of your team. They can help you express your feelings about your care to the team. Treatment of other health problems may be improved if they are aware of and involved in your cancer care.

Cancer treatment

There is often more than one treatment option, including clinical trials. Clinical trials study the safety and effectiveness of investigational treatments. The treatment that you and your care team agree on should be described in the treatment plan, along with known side effects.

Keep in mind that your treatment plan may change. Testing may provide new information. How well the treatment is working may change the plan. Or you may change your mind about treatment. Any of these changes may require a new treatment plan.

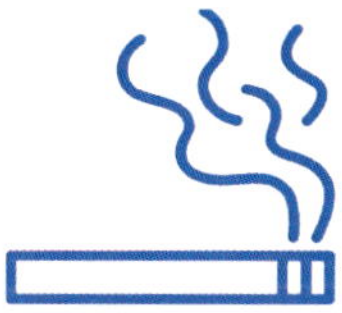

If you smoke or vape, seek help to quit

If you smoke or vape, it's important to quit. Smoking can limit how well cancer treatment works. Smoking and vaping can also increase the risk of lung problems during and after chemotherapy. They also increase your chances of developing other cancers.

Nicotine is the chemical in tobacco that makes you want to keep smoking. Nicotine withdrawal is challenging for most people who smoke. The stress of having cancer may make it even harder to quit. If you smoke, ask your care team about resources and programs that can help you quit.

For online support, try these websites:

- SmokeFree.gov
- BeTobaccoFree.gov
- CDC.gov/tobacco

Stress and symptom control

Anxiety and depression are common in people with cancer. At your cancer center, cancer navigators, social workers, and others can help. Help may include support groups, talk therapy, exercising, spending time with loved ones, or medication.

You may be unemployed or miss work during treatment. Or, you may have little or no health insurance. Talk to your treatment team about work, insurance, or money concerns. They will include information in the treatment plan to help you manage the costs of care.

For more information, see the *NCCN Guidelines for Patients: Distress During Cancer Care* at NCCN.org/patientguidelines and on the NCCN Patient Guides for Cancer app for more information.

Supportive care

Supportive care aims to relieve the symptoms of cancer or the side effects of cancer treatment. It can help relieve discomfort and improve quality of life. Supportive care may be given alone or with cancer treatment.

Key points

- Cervical cancer is most often diagnosed by cervical biopsy. Samples of cervical tissue are removed and tested for dysplasia and cancer.
- A cone biopsy may be used to gather more information after a cervical biopsy or to treat early cervical cancer. It involves removing a cone-shaped portion of the cervix.
- Blood tests provide helpful information about your general health and the health of your liver, kidneys, and other organs before treatment.
- Imaging helps determine the extent of the cancer before treatment. Initial imaging may include CT, MRI, PET, or transvaginal ultrasound.
- A cystoscopy and/or proctoscopy under anesthesia may be needed to look for signs of cancer in the bladder and bowel.
- Quitting smoking can lead to better cancer treatment outcomes. Help is available when you are ready to stop smoking.

Questions to ask

- Which imaging tests do I need?
- What are the newest options to help me quit smoking?
- What choices do I have for preserving my fertility?

3
Staging

The results of imaging and other testing are used to determine the stage (extent) of the cancer. Your treatment options will depend on the cancer stage.

The International Federation of Gynecology and Obstetrics (FIGO) system is used to stage cervical cancer. There are four main stages in the FIGO system: I (1), II (2), III (3), and IV (4). The stages are broken down into sub-stages that have letters and may also have a number.

The following information is used to stage the cancer in the FIGO system:

- The size or extent/depth of the tumor
- Whether any lymph nodes have cancer
- Whether the cancer has spread to involve nearby organs, like the bladder or rectum
- Whether the cancer has spread (metastasized) to distant organs such as the liver, lungs, and/or bone

The stages of cervical cancer

The stages are explained and pictured on the following pages. If the cancer grows or spreads, the stage doesn't change.

In general, people with earlier cancer stages have better outcomes, but not always. Some people will do better than expected for their stage, and some will do worse.

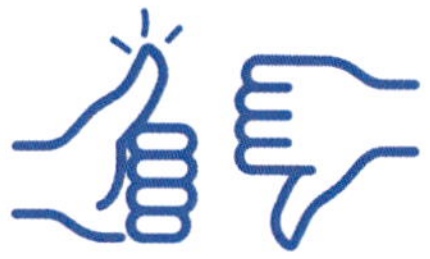

Let us know what you think!

Please take a moment to complete an online survey about the NCCN Guidelines for Patients.
NCCN.org/patients/response

Stage 1A cervical cancer

The cancer is 5 millimeters (mm) or smaller. 5 mm is about the size of a standard pencil eraser.

- **Cancers 3 mm or smaller are stage 1A1.**
- **Cancers between 3 and 5 mm are stage 1A2.**

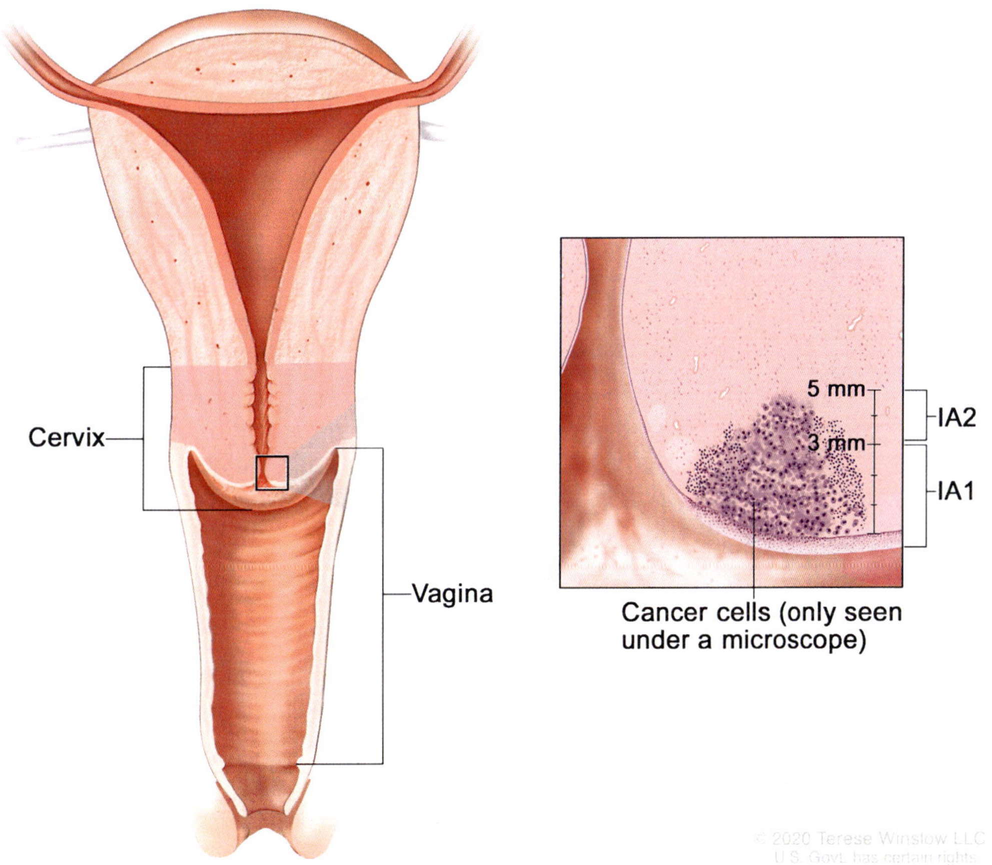

Stage 1B1 cervical cancer

The cancer is larger than 5 mm but smaller than 2 centimeters (cm).

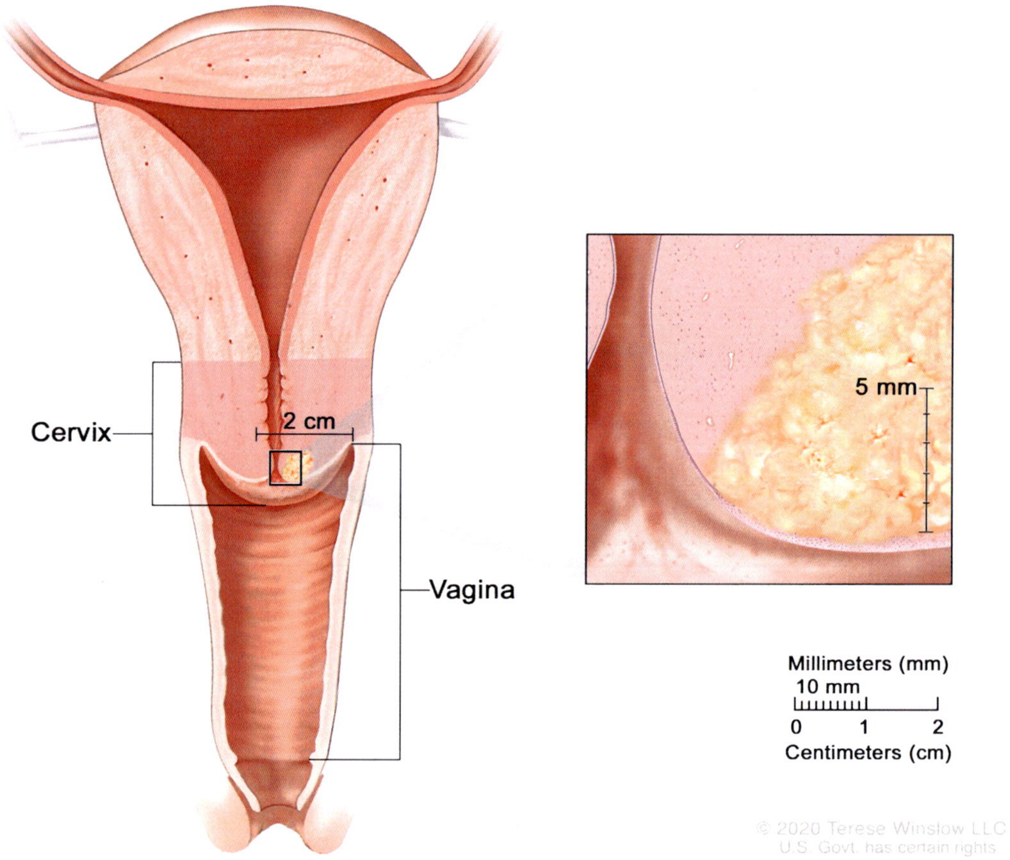

Stage 1B2 and 1B3 cervical cancer

The cancer is only in the cervix. In stage 1B2, the cancer is between 2 and 4 cm. In stage 1B3, the cancer is larger than 4 cm.

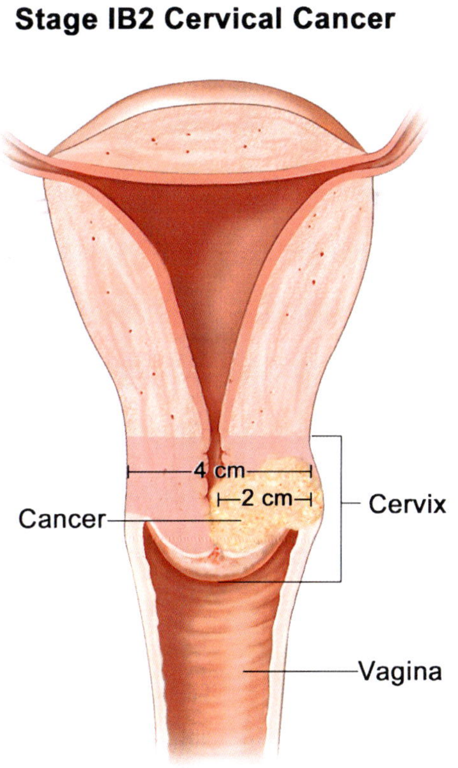

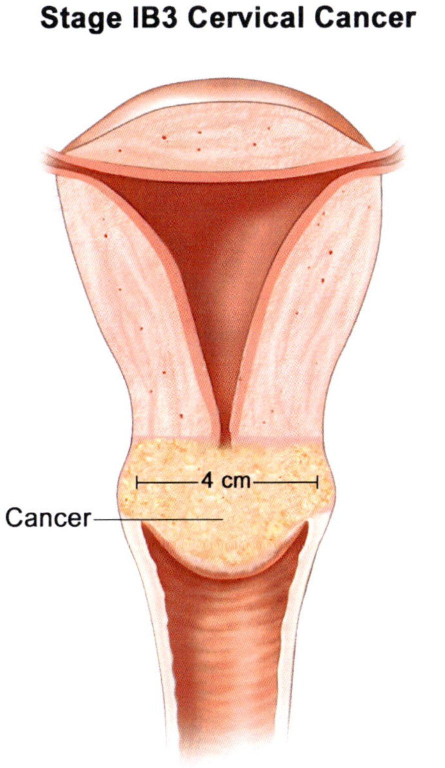

Stage 2 cervical cancer

The cancer has grown beyond the cervix. If the cancer has grown into the upper vagina, the stage is 2A. Stage 2A1 cancers are 4 cm or smaller. Stage 2A2 cancers are larger than 4 cm. Stage 2B cancer has grown into the parametrium. The parametrium is the fat and connective tissue that surrounds the cervix and uterus.

Stages IIA1 and IIA2 Cervical Cancer

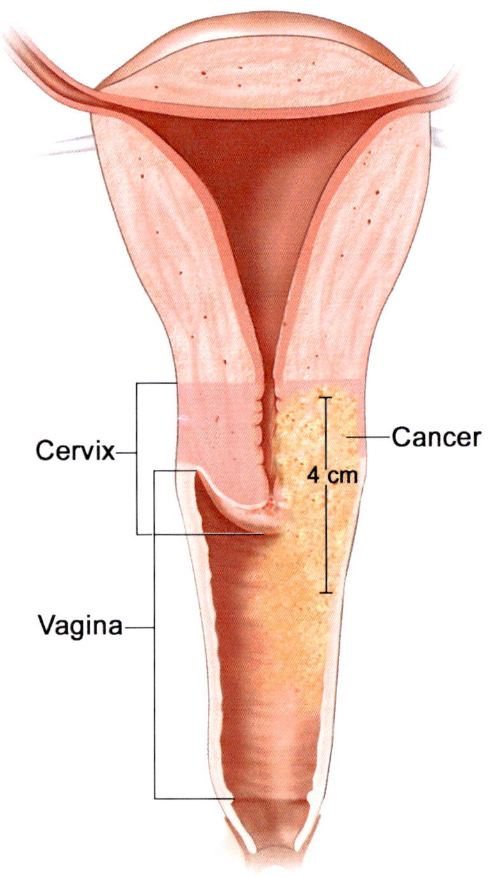

Stage IIB Cervical Cancer

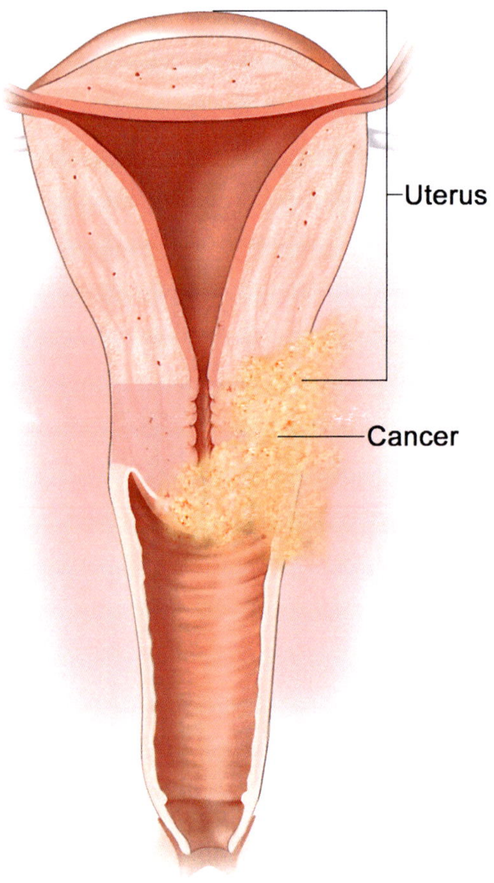

Stage 3A cervical cancer

The cancer has grown into the lower third of the vagina.

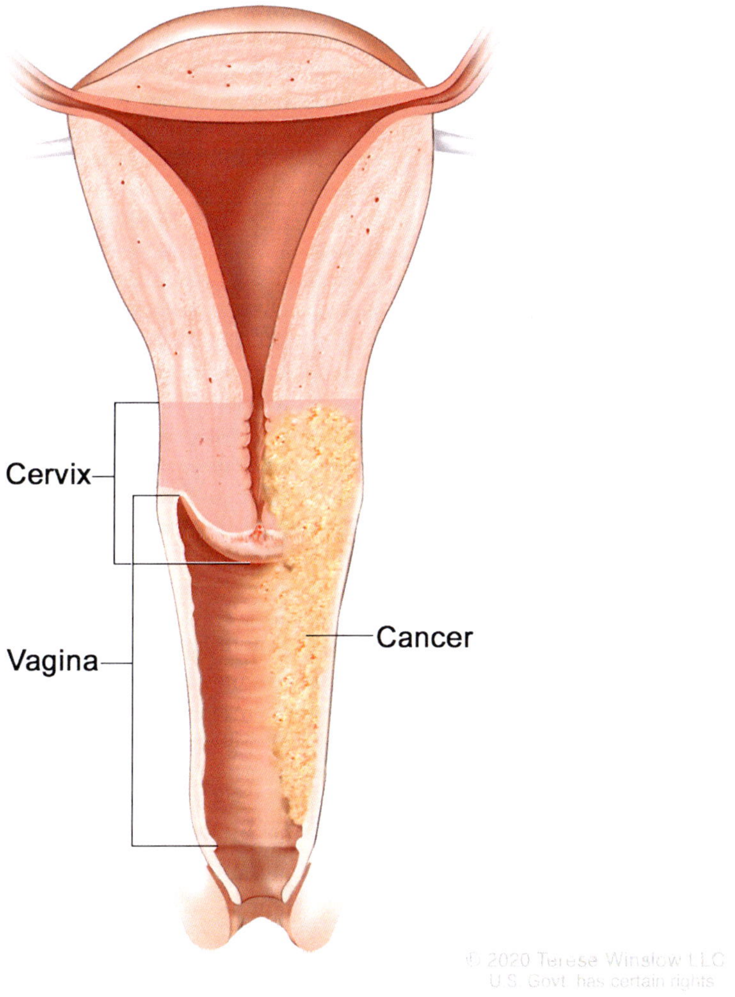

Stage 3B cervical cancer

The cancer has grown into the pelvic wall and/or has caused kidney swelling or dysfunction.

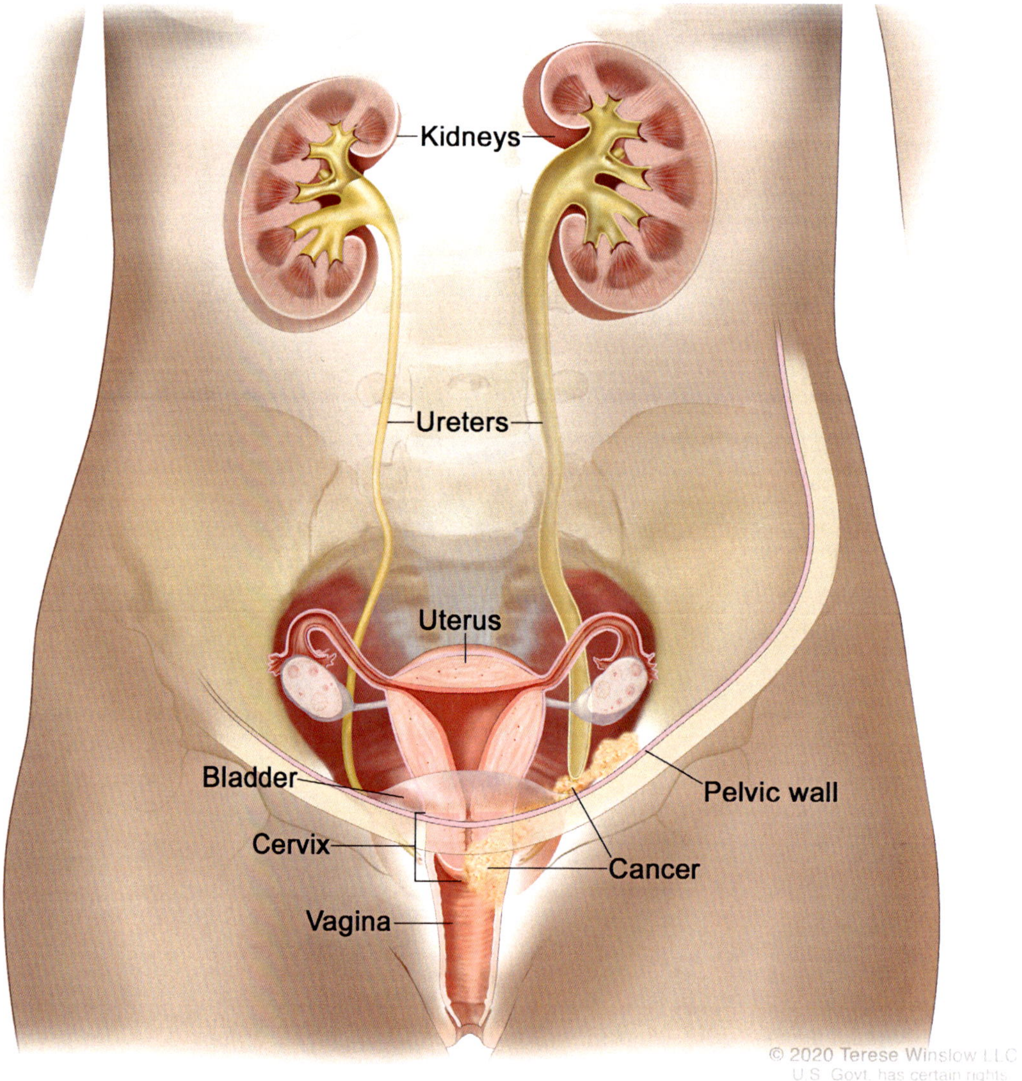

Stage 3C cervical cancer

There is cancer in lymph nodes near the cervix (pelvic lymph nodes) and/ or in lymph nodes in the abdomen, called the para-aortic lymph nodes.

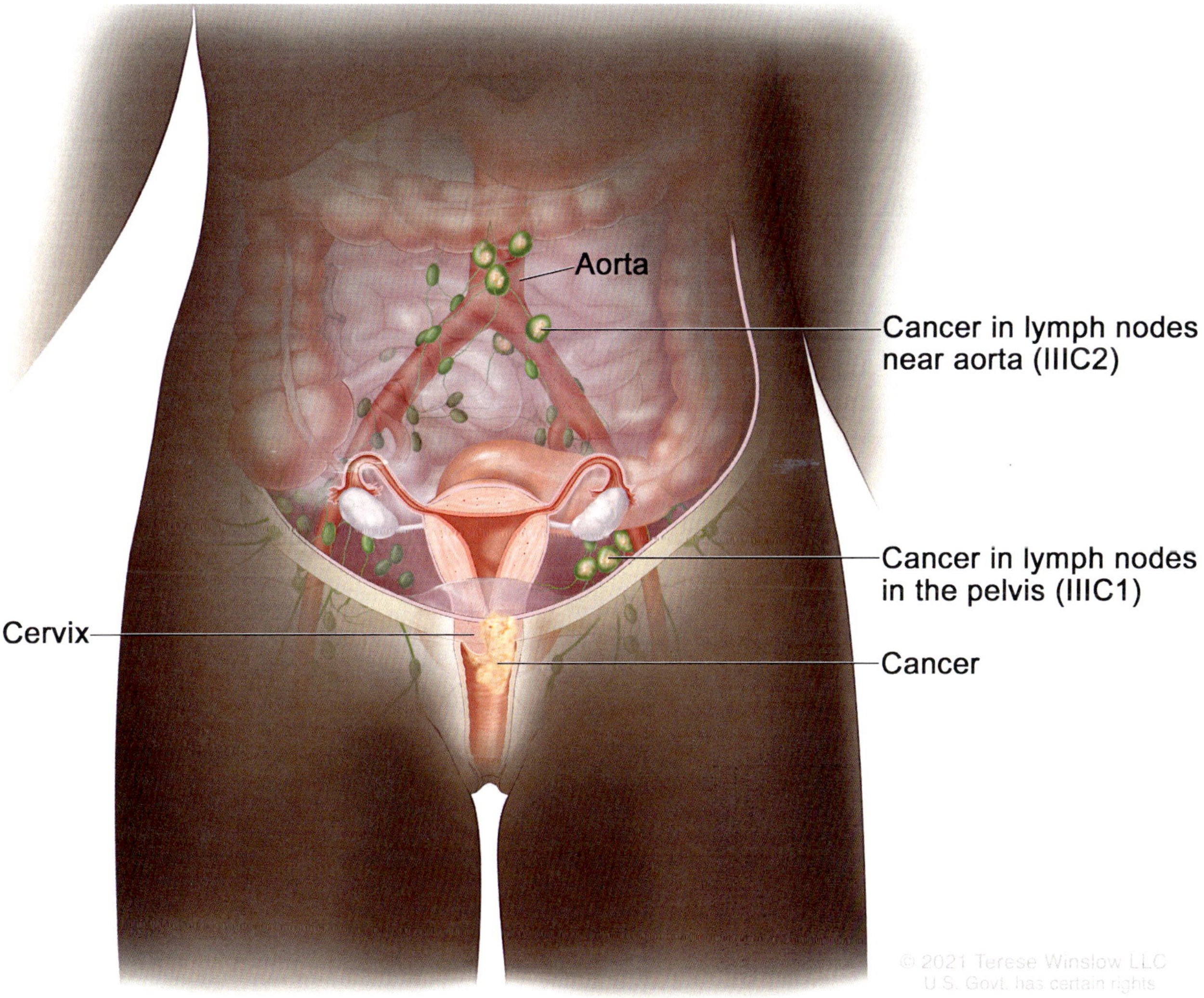

Stage 4A cervical cancer

The cancer has spread to nearby organs, such as the bladder or rectum.

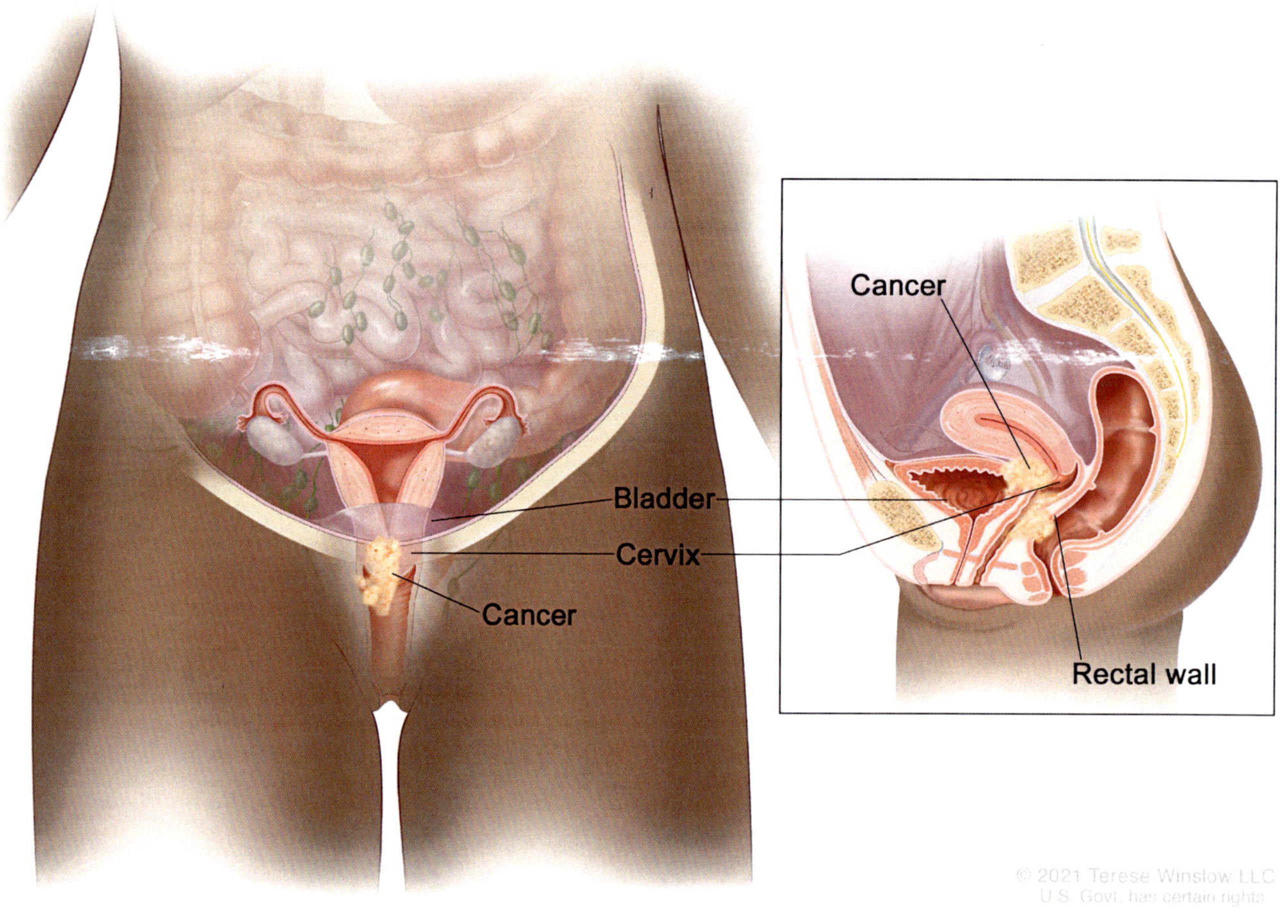

Stage 4B cervical cancer

The cancer is metastatic. It has spread to the liver, lungs, abdomen, bone, or other distant sites or lymph nodes.

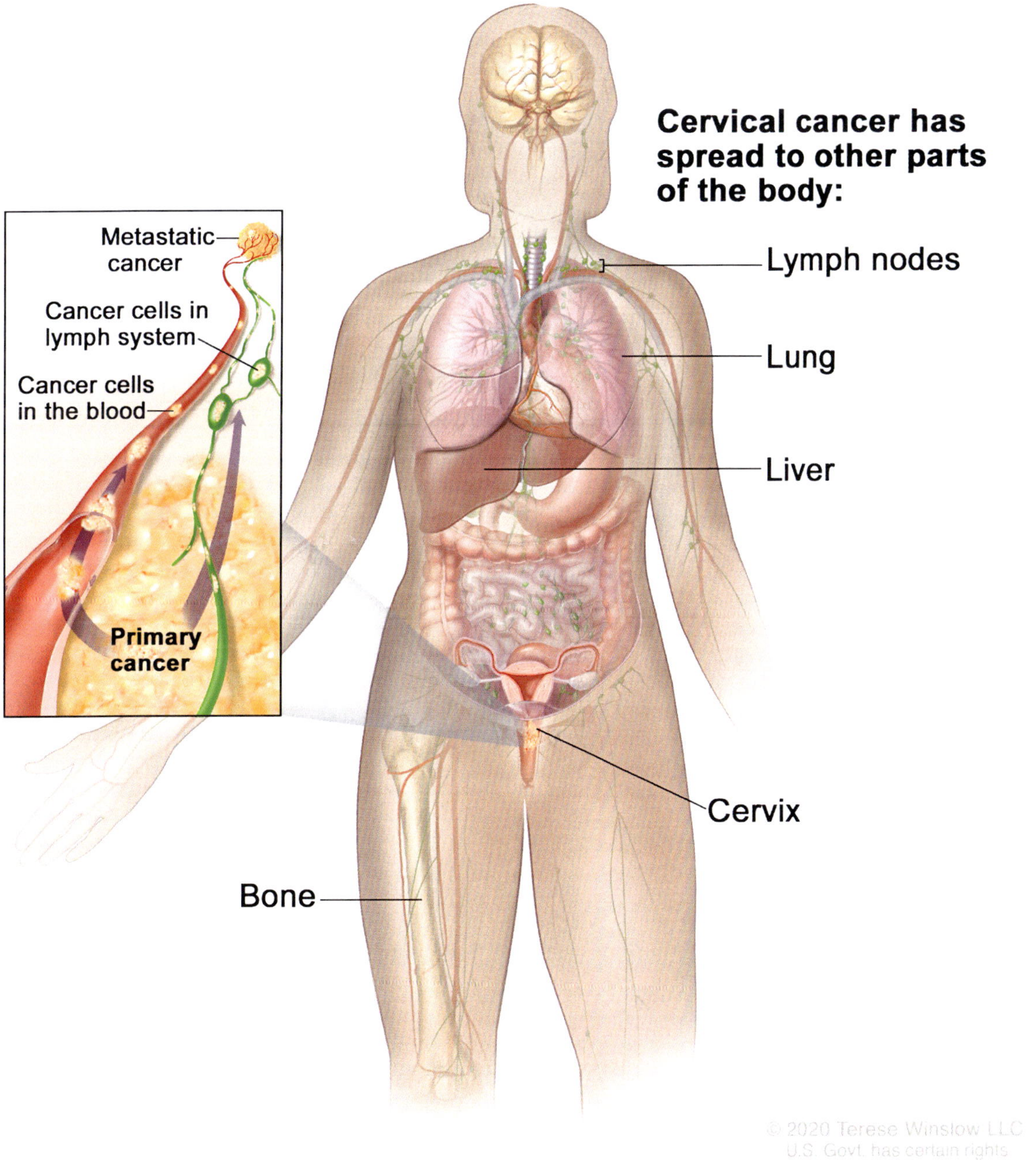

Key points

- The stage is a rating of the extent of the cancer before any treatment is given. It is used to determine your treatment options.
- The International Federation of Gynecology and Obstetrics (FIGO) system is used to stage cervical cancer. There are 4 main stages in the FIGO system: I (1), II (2), III (3), and IV (4).

Questions to ask

- What stage is the cancer?
- If the cancer spreads, does the stage change?

4

Types of treatment

In this chapter, the main treatments for cervical cancer are described. Your treatment options will depend on the extent of the cancer and other factors.

Surgery

In most cases, surgery for cervical cancer involves removing the entire cervix. Removing only a portion may be an option for the earliest stage of cervical cancer.

While removing the cervix can sometimes be performed through the vagina, a long incision (cut) through the abdomen is usually needed. When performed through the abdomen, the approach is known as laparotomy.

Minimally invasive (also called laparoscopic) surgery involves making only a few small cuts into your body. There is usually less pain and scarring compared to surgery that uses a larger cut through the abdomen. The time it takes to recover is also usually shorter.

Cone biopsy

Cone biopsy involves removing a cone-shaped section of the cervix that includes tissue from both the ectocervix and endocervix. It is a recommended treatment option for some small cervical cancers. See *Chapter 2: Testing for cervical cancer* for more information on cone biopsy.

Trachelectomy

Trachelectomy is a fertility-sparing surgery that removes the cervix, and sometimes other tissues.

In a simple trachelectomy, only the cervix is removed. In a radical trachelectomy, about 2 centimeters (a little less than an inch) of vaginal tissue is also removed. Both types can be performed either through the vagina or the abdomen.

The uterus and ovaries are left in place during trachelectomy, allowing for the possibility of natural pregnancy in the future.

Hysterectomy

Hysterectomy is surgery to remove the uterus (including the cervix). Depending on the type of hysterectomy performed, other nearby tissues may also be removed.

A Type A (simple) hysterectomy removes only the uterus (including the cervix). It's most commonly used for very early cervical cancers. Type A hysterectomy can be performed through the vagina, through the abdomen, or using a minimally invasive approach.

A Type B radical hysterectomy removes the uterus (including the cervix), some connective tissue that holds the cervix in place, and about a half inch or less of the vagina. Modified radical hysterectomy is performed through the abdomen.

A Type C1 radical hysterectomy removes the uterus (including the cervix), much of the connective tissue that holds the cervix in place, and the top quarter or third of the vagina.

Radical hysterectomy is performed through the abdomen.

There are other differences between these procedures. If surgery is planned, your surgeon will explain the procedure recommended for you in detail.

Will my ovaries be removed?

The ovaries may or may not be removed during hysterectomy. In premenopausal people, surgically removing the ovaries causes a sudden drop in estrogen in the body. This is called surgical menopause.

Symptoms include hot flashes, sleeping problems, night sweats, weight gain, and changes in mood. It's also common for the lining of the vagina to become thin, dry, and inflamed. This is called vaginal atrophy.

Long-term risks of not having enough estrogen include heart disease and weakened bones (osteoporosis). If hysterectomy is being considered, ask your provider about the benefits and risks of keeping your ovaries.

Checking lymph nodes for cancer

Lymph nodes are bean-shaped glands that help the body fight infection and disease. During surgery for cervical cancer, lymph nodes may be removed in order to be tested for cancer. This is called lymph node dissection or lymphadenectomy.

Testing the removed nodes helps determine the extent (spread) of the cancer. Removing lymph nodes can also help limit the spread of cancer cells through lymph.

The closest lymph nodes to the cervix are the pelvic nodes. Cervical cancer generally spreads to these nodes first. Lymph nodes in the abdomen, called the para-aortic nodes, are also sometimes removed.

In order to identify and remove the lymph node(s) most likely to contain cancer, a sentinel lymph node biopsy may be performed. This involves injecting a special dye or a radioactive substance into the cervix near the cancer. Lymph nodes containing the dye or substance can be seen using a special camera. These are the sentinel nodes.

Staging before surgery

A hysterectomy generally isn't the first treatment for more advanced cervical cancers. So in order to know how far the cancer has spread, lymph nodes may be removed from your pelvis or abdomen and tested before any treatment is given. Knowing whether the nodes contain cancer helps your provider make the most informed recommendations for your care.

A minimally invasive approach is typically used to access and remove the lymph nodes. This is called laparoscopic surgical staging.

External beam radiation therapy

Radiation therapy uses high-energy waves similar to x-rays to kill cancer cells. In external beam radiation therapy (EBRT), a large machine aims radiation at the cancer site. The radiation passes through skin and other tissue to reach the tumor and nearby lymph nodes. EBRT is given in small doses, called fractions.

An advanced type of EBRT called intensity-modulated radiation therapy (IMRT) is often used to treat cervical cancer. IMRT allows a high dose of radiation to reach the tumor while limiting the amount that reaches the surrounding normal tissue. With IMRT it is possible to reduce radiation to important nearby organs and structures, such as the bowel, bladder, external genitalia, and hip joints. This can help reduce treatment-related side effects.

Stereotactic body radiation therapy (SBRT) is a highly specialized type of EBRT used to treat metastatic cervical cancer. High doses of radiation are delivered to tumors in the liver, lungs, or bone using very precise beams. Treatment is typically delivered in 5 or fewer sessions.

Common side effects during the 5 to 6 weeks of EBRT include fatigue, skin redness and irritation, diarrhea, nausea, and frequent or painful urination. Most of these side effects come on slowly during treatment and gradually decrease afterward.

Early menopause

When the ovaries are included in the radiation field, it causes premature (early) menopause. The symptoms are similar to those caused by surgical menopause, as described above.

External beam radiation therapy

A large machine aims radiation at the tumor, passing through skin and other tissue to reach it.

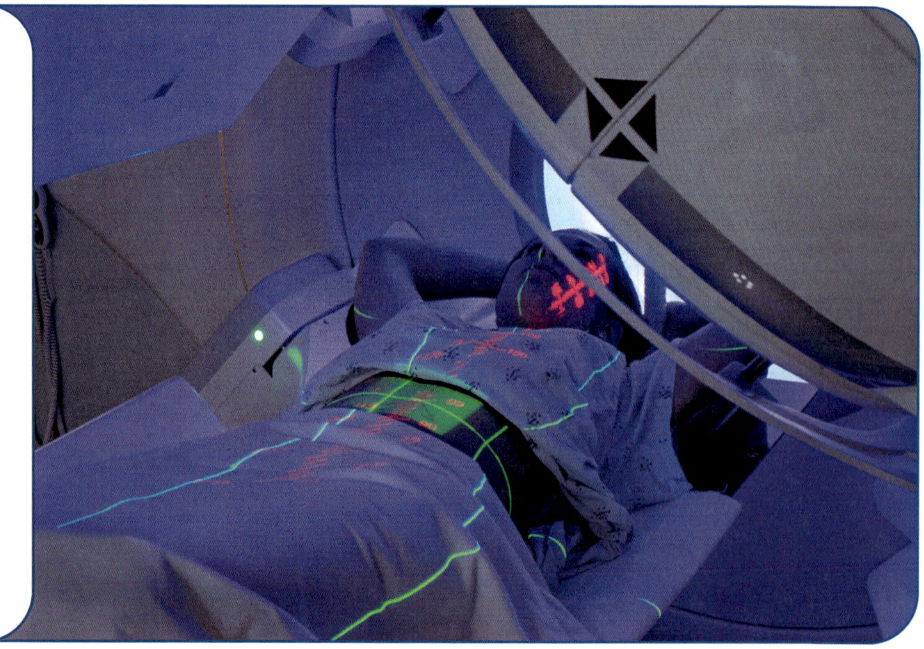

Ovarian transposition is a surgery that moves one or both ovaries out of the range of the radiation beam. This procedure may be an option if you are premenopausal and the cancer is a squamous cell carcinoma (the most common type of cervical cancer).

Otherwise, your provider may suggest the use of menopausal hormone therapy (MHT) after radiation therapy has completed. Hormone therapy for menopause helps lessen some of the side effects of radiation-induced menopause. This approach used to be called hormone replacement therapy or HRT. See *Chapter 7: Survivorship* for more information.

Radiation therapy for cervical cancer can also have long-term and serious side effects on fertility, sexual health, and bowel and bladder function.

What to expect

A planning session, called simulation, is needed before EBRT begins. You will first be placed in the treatment position. You will be asked to lie on your back and stay very still. You may get fitted for a prop to help you stay still during the radiation sessions.

Pictures of the cancer site(s) will be obtained with a CT scan. Using the CT images and sophisticated computer software, your radiation oncologist will make a treatment plan. The plan will specify the radiation dose(s) and the number of sessions you will need.

There will be several days between the time of simulation and the beginning of your treatment sessions. This allows sufficient time for careful treatment planning, dose calculation, and quality assurance.

During treatment, you will lie on a table as you did for simulation. Devices may be used to keep you from moving. This helps to target the tumor. Ink marks (tattoos) on your skin will help position your body accurately for daily treatments. The technician will be operating the machine from an adjacent room. You will be able to see, hear, and speak with them at all times. You will not see, hear, or feel the radiation. One session can take less than 10 minutes.

Chemoradiation

EBRT and chemotherapy are often used together during the same time period to treat cervical cancer. This treatment strategy is called chemoradiation. Chemoradiation is recommended for most locally advanced cervical cancers. These cancers have grown beyond the cervix but haven't spread to the liver, lungs, or bones.

As part of chemoradiation, there are typically 5 EBRT treatment sessions per week for 5 to 6 weeks. Chemotherapy with cisplatin is typically given on a 7-day cycle (once weekly) during this time. An immunotherapy treatment called pembrolizumab (Keytruda) may also be given with chemotherapy.

Brachytherapy

Also known as internal radiation therapy, brachytherapy involves treatment with radioactive material placed inside the body. Brachytherapy allows a high dose of radiation to be targeted at the tumor while limiting the amount delivered to surrounding normal tissue.

During brachytherapy, instruments are placed into the cervix, uterus, and vagina. A radioactive material then travels into the instruments that have been placed in the body. This method is known as intracavitary brachytherapy. Sometimes, additional instruments (catheters, or thin hollow tubes) are placed in the tumor itself or in tissues next to the tumor (interstitial brachytherapy).

For the treatment of cervical cancer, intracavitary brachytherapy is most often used. Interstitial brachytherapy is a specialized technique that is used for more advanced cancers that involve the parametrium. It is best performed at cancer centers with experience in this method.

Brachytherapy for cervical cancer may be given in short bursts, called high dose-rate (HDR) brachytherapy, or in long bursts, called low dose-rate (LDR) brachytherapy. Most centers currently use HDR brachytherapy. Treatment is typically given in 3 to 5 sessions over 2 weeks.

For those receiving treatment primarily with radiation and systemic therapy, a device called an applicator is inserted into the uterus through the vagina. A "tandem and ring" applicator is commonly used for HDR brachytherapy. The tandem is a long, thin tube that extends into the uterus. The ring is a hollow circle that stays in the vagina, pressed against the cervix. A tandem and ovoid applicator uses hollow, rounded capsules instead of a ring. General anesthesia or deep sedation is often required, especially for the first applicator placement.

The applicator is placed to align with the tissue targeted for treatment. Often, an imaging technique (MRI or CT) is used to guide placement of the applicator. These images are used to design the brachytherapy treatment plan. The applicator is connected to a brachytherapy machine. A radiation source travels from the machine through the hollow tubes and into the applicator. Treatment takes about 10 minutes.

Sometimes brachytherapy is given as treatments over a couple of days. In this case, the instruments are placed and left in the body until all the treatments have been given (1 to 2 days). You will need to remain in bed until treatment is complete so that the instruments don't move.

Brachytherapy is typically started in the final week or right after completing EBRT. Shrinking the tumor with EBRT first allows for better placement of the brachytherapy applicators. Treatment with both types of radiation therapy can be completed within 7 to 8 weeks.

Side effects

The side effects of brachytherapy are similar to those of EBRT and include:

- Skin irritation near treatment area
- Tiredness (fatigue)
- Soreness in your pelvic area
- Difficulty urinating or painful urination
- Softer bowel movements or diarrhea
- Increased vaginal discharge

Systemic therapy

Systemic therapy is treatment with substances that travel in the bloodstream, reaching cells throughout the body. Chemotherapy, targeted therapy, and immunotherapy are types of systemic therapy.

Platinum-based chemotherapy is the most commonly used systemic therapy for cervical cancer. Cisplatin is generally preferred, but carboplatin may be used instead if needed. Targeted therapy and immunotherapy are newer types of systemic therapy.

Most systemic therapies are slowly infused into your bloodstream through a vein. Infusions are often given in cycles of treatment days followed by days of rest. This allows your body to recover between cycles.

Common side effects of systemic therapy include:

- Loss of appetite
- Nausea
- Vomiting
- Mouth sores
- Hair loss
- Fatigue
- Increased risk of infection
- Bleeding or bruising easily
- Nerve damage (neuropathy)

Cisplatin can damage the kidneys. People whose kidneys don't work well may receive a different chemotherapy drug. Cisplatin can also cause ringing in the ears and hearing problems or loss.

Ask your care team for a list of side effects of each systemic therapy you are receiving.

Clinical trials

A clinical trial is a type of medical research study. After being developed and tested in a lab, potential new ways of fighting cancer need to be studied in people.

If found to be safe and effective in a clinical trial, a drug, device, or treatment approach may be approved by the U.S. Food and Drug Administration (FDA).

Everyone with cancer should carefully consider all of the treatment options available for their cancer type, including standard treatments and clinical trials. Talk to your doctor about whether a clinical trial may make sense for you.

Phases

Most cancer clinical trials focus on treatment and are done in phases.

- **Phase 1** trials study the safety and side effects of an investigational drug or treatment approach.
- **Phase 2** trials study how well the drug or approach works against a specific type of cancer.
- **Phase 3** trials test the drug or approach against a standard treatment. If the results are good, it may be approved by the FDA.

- **Phase 4** trials study the safety and benefit of an FDA-approved treatment.

Who can enroll?

It depends on the clinical trial's rules, called eligibility criteria. The rules may be about age, cancer type and stage, treatment history, or general health. They ensure that participants are alike in specific ways and that the trial is as safe as possible for the participants.

Informed consent

Clinical trials are managed by a research team. This group of experts will review the study with you in detail, including its purpose and the risks and benefits of joining. All of this information is also provided in an informed consent form. Read the form carefully and ask questions before signing it. Take time to discuss it with people you trust. Keep in mind that you can leave and seek treatment outside of the clinical trial at any time.

Will I get a placebo?

Placebos (inactive versions of real medicines) are almost never used alone in cancer clinical trials. It is common to receive either a placebo with a standard treatment, or a new drug with a standard treatment. You will be informed, verbally and in writing, if a placebo is part of a clinical trial before you enroll.

Are clinical trials free?

There is no fee to enroll in a clinical trial. The study sponsor pays for research-related costs, including the study drug. But you may need to pay for other services, like transportation or childcare, due to extra appointments. During the trial, you will continue to receive standard cancer care. This care is often covered by insurance.

Finding a clinical trial

In the United States

NCCN Cancer Centers
NCCN.org/cancercenters

The National Cancer Institute (NCI)
cancer.gov/about-cancer/treatment/clinical-trials/search

Worldwide

The U.S. National Library of Medicine (NLM)
clinicaltrials.gov

Need help finding a clinical trial?

NCI's Cancer Information Service (CIS)
1.800.4.CANCER (1.800.422.6237)
cancer.gov/contact

Key points

- Hysterectomy is surgery that removes the uterus, including the cervix. Some of the vagina and cervical connective tissue may also be removed. The ovaries may be removed or left in place. Removing them causes early menopause.
- Trachelectomy is surgery that removes the cervix. It is a type of fertility-sparing surgery. The upper part of the vagina may also be removed.
- Radiation therapy uses high-energy x-rays to kill cancer cells. In EBRT, a large machine aims radiation at the cancer site.
- Brachytherapy involves treatment with radioactive material placed inside the body. It delivers a high dose of radiation directly to the tumor.
- Platinum-based chemotherapy is the most commonly used systemic therapy for cervical cancer.
- EBRT and platinum-based chemotherapy given during the same time period is a treatment strategy called chemoradiation.
- Clinical trials provide access to investigational treatments that may, in time, be approved by the FDA.

Questions to ask

- What are the side effects of systemic therapy?
- What are the side effects of brachytherapy and EBRT?
- Should I consider a clinical trial?

5

Treatment for common types

This chapter presents recommended treatment options for the most common types of cervical cancer. Surgery is usually recommended for early-stage cancers, while most locally advanced cancers are treated with chemoradiation.

This section applies to the following types of cervical cancer:

- Squamous cell carcinoma
- Adenocarcinoma
- Adenosquamous carcinoma

Treatment is based on the cancer stage. The stage describes how far the cancer has (likely) spread based on imaging and other testing.

A risk factor that guides treatment for cervical cancer is whether there are cancer cells in blood vessels or lymph vessels near the tumor. This is called **lymphovascular space invasion (LVSI)**. Cancers with LVSI are more likely to spread to nearby lymph nodes. Removing and testing lymph nodes near the cancer will be part of your care.

Fertility-sparing treatment

Surgical treatment for early-stage cervical cancer often involves hysterectomy. Carrying a pregnancy isn't possible after the uterus is removed. If the cancer hasn't spread beyond the cervix, fertility-sparing treatment may be an option (if desired).

This approach involves surgery that doesn't remove the uterus or ovaries, allowing you the option of natural pregnancy in the future. If fertility-sparing treatment is being considered, ask your provider about getting the opinion of a reproductive endocrinologist. These are doctors that specialize in fertility.

Keep in mind that a fertility-sparing approach isn't recommended for some uncommon types of cervical cancer.

Stage 1A1

Cone biopsy is recommended for stage 1A1 cancers **without known LVSI**. If the results are good, treatment is over. If the results suggest that the cancer wasn't fully removed, you may have another cone biopsy, or your provider may recommend trachelectomy.

For stage 1A1 cancers **with LVSI**, treatment with either cone biopsy or radical trachelectomy is recommended. Lymph nodes in the pelvis will also be removed and tested.

Stage 1A2

Cone biopsy is an option for some small (no larger than 2 cm) stage 1A2 cancers **without LVSI** that also meet other low-risk criteria. Lymph nodes in the pelvis will also be removed and tested.

For stage 1A2 cancers **with LVSI**, treatment with either cone biopsy or radical trachelectomy is recommended. Lymph nodes in the pelvis will also be removed and tested.

Stage 1B1

Cone biopsy is an option for some small (no larger than 2 cm) stage 1B1 cancers without LVSI that also meet other low-risk criteria. Lymph nodes in the pelvis will also be removed and tested.

For stage 1B1 cancers that don't meet the criteria for cone biopsy, radical trachelectomy is recommended. Lymph nodes in the pelvis, and possibly in the abdomen, will also be removed and tested.

Stage 1B2

Because most research on fertility-sparing surgery applies to smaller tumors, it isn't performed often for stage 1B2 cancers. Abdominal surgery is generally preferred.

Results of surgery and next steps

If no cancer is found in the removed lymph nodes or in tissues outside the cervix, EBRT may be needed next.

Your provider will consider the tumor size, whether there is LVSI, and other factors to decide if EBRT is a good choice for you. If you don't need radiation therapy, observation will begin. If radiation is planned, platinum chemotherapy may be given during the same time period. This is called chemoradiation.

If cancer is found in any of the lymph nodes removed during surgery, or in any tissues outside the cervix, chemoradiation is recommended. Vaginal brachytherapy may be given in addition to chemoradiation.

Fertility-sparing treatment

Fertility-sparing treatment may be an option, if desired, for some stage 1 cancers. This approach involves surgery that does not remove the uterus or ovaries, allowing you the option of natural pregnancy in the future.

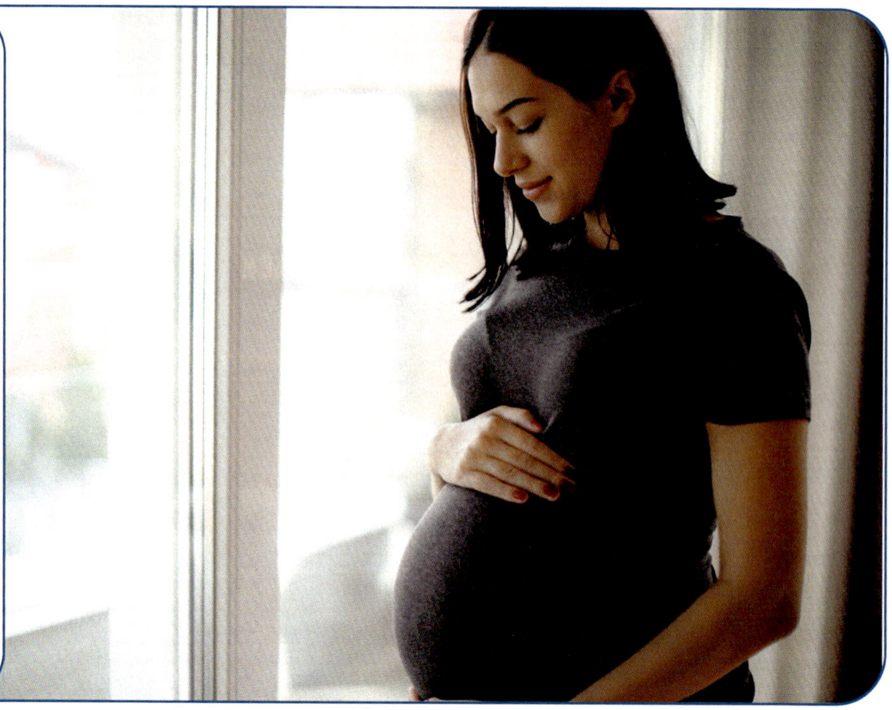

Early-stage cancer

This section describes **non–fertility-sparing** treatment for:

- Cancers that are only in the cervix (stage 1)
- Cancers that have spread to the upper vagina (stage 2A)

Stage 1A1

Stage 1A1 cancers are typically diagnosed by cone biopsy. **If no cancer or pre-cancer is found** at the margins (edges) of the removed tissue, a Type A hysterectomy is recommended next. For cancers with LVSI, nearby lymph nodes will be removed during surgery and tested.

If you aren't a candidate for surgery, recommended next steps include:

- Observation (for cancers without LVSI)
- EBRT and brachytherapy (for cancers with LVSI)

If cancer or pre-cancer is found at the margins of the tissue removed during cone biopsy, you might have another cone biopsy to confirm the stage. If pre-cancer cells (also called dysplasia) are found at the margins of this biopsy, a Type A hysterectomy is recommended.

If cancer cells (also called carcinoma) are found, a Type B radical hysterectomy is recommended. Nearby lymph nodes will be removed during either type of surgery. Depending on the results of surgery, you may need more treatment. See the next page for information.

If you aren't a candidate for surgery, recommended next steps include:

- Brachytherapy, and maybe also EBRT (for cancers without LVSI)
- Brachytherapy and EBRT (for cancers with LVSI)

Stages 1A2 and 1B1

For **low-risk cancers**, a Type A hysterectomy is recommended. The surgeon will remove nearby lymph nodes during surgery. Features of low-risk cancers include:

- **No LVSI**
- No cancer found in cone biopsy margins
- The tumor is a common type of cervical cancer
- The tumor is 2 cm or smaller and not very deep
- No signs of cancer spread in the body

For all other stage 1A2 and 1B1 cancers, a Type C1 radical hysterectomy is recommended. The surgeon will remove lymph nodes from the pelvis, and maybe from the abdomen, during surgery.

If surgery isn't an option, treatment with EBRT and brachytherapy is recommended. Platinum chemotherapy might also be given during the same time period.

Stage 1B2 and 2A1

A Type C1 radical hysterectomy is recommended for stage 1B2 and 2A1 cancers. The surgeon will remove lymph nodes from the pelvis, and maybe from the abdomen, during surgery.

If surgery isn't an option, treatment with EBRT and brachytherapy is recommended. Platinum chemotherapy might also be given during the same time period.

Stage 1B3 and 2A2

These cancers may be treated as early-stage (with surgery) or as locally advanced (with chemoradiation and brachytherapy). If treatment with chemoradiation and brachytherapy is planned, you may have chemotherapy first. This is called induction chemotherapy.

If surgery is planned, a Type C1 radical hysterectomy is recommended. The surgeon will remove lymph nodes from your pelvis, and maybe from your abdomen.

Do I need more treatment?

After surgery, the pathologic (surgical) stage of the cancer is determined by examining the removed tissue.

The following information applies to the stages below, as determined by surgery:

- Stage 1
- Stage 2A

If testing finds no cancer in tissue beyond the cervix or in lymph nodes removed during surgery, you may still need more treatment. EBRT is recommended for cancers with risk factors. Your provider will consider the tumor size, whether there is LVSI, and other factors to determine if radiation therapy is a good choice for you.

If EBRT is planned, platinum chemotherapy may be given during the same time period. This is called chemoradiation.

If cancer is found in any of the removed lymph nodes, or in any tissues outside the cervix, treatment with chemoradiation is recommended. Vaginal brachytherapy may be given in addition to EBRT and platinum chemotherapy.

Locally advanced cancer

Cervical cancer that has grown beyond the cervix but hasn't spread to the liver, lungs, or bones is described as locally advanced. Locally advanced cancers are not metastatic.

The information in this section applies to the following stages:

- Stage 2B
- Stage 3
- Stage 4A

Checking lymph nodes

Locally advanced cancers are more likely to have spread to lymph nodes than early-stage cancers. You may have extra imaging to look for lymph nodes with cancer.

Another approach is to surgically remove and test lymph nodes before any treatment is given. A minimally invasive method is typically used to access and remove the lymph nodes. This is called surgical staging.

If surgical staging is performed, lymph nodes in the abdomen (para-aortic nodes) are typically removed. Pelvic lymph nodes may or may not be removed.

Treatment

Treatment with chemoradiation and brachytherapy is recommended for most locally advanced cervical cancers. Depending on the cancer stage, pembrolizumab (Keytruda) may also be given with the platinum chemotherapy you receive for chemoradiation.

Before chemoradiation begins, you may have chemotherapy first with carboplatin and paclitaxel together. This is called induction chemotherapy.

If any lymph nodes in the abdomen are known or suspected to have cancer, the radiation will be given to a larger treatment area that includes these nodes as well.

It's important to take care of yourself during cancer care. Try to eat nutritious foods, drink plenty of fluids, exercise, and do things that make you feel energized.

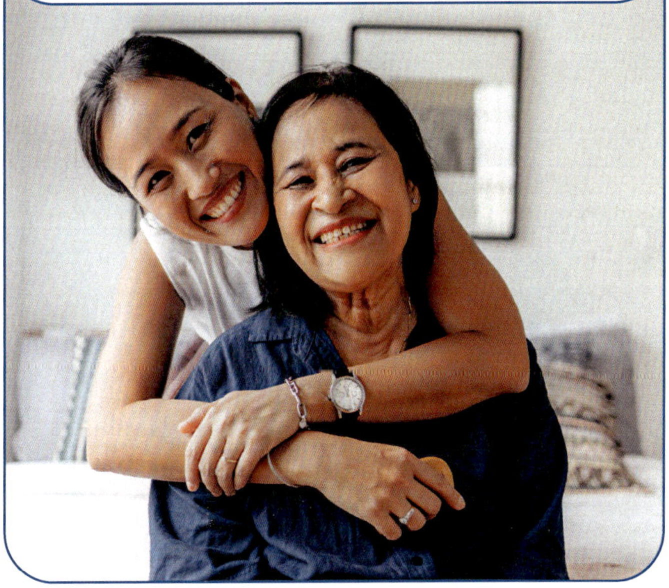

Surveillance

After finishing treatment, you will have testing to look for early signs of possible recurrence. This is known as surveillance. The information that follows applies to surveillance for common types of cervical cancer and for small cell neuroendocrine carcinoma of the cervix (NECC).

Physical exams

Physical exams performed by your oncologist are an important part of surveillance, especially in the first 5 years after treatment. At these follow-up visits, tell your provider about any changes in your health. Such changes include new or worsening symptoms and other health conditions or concerns.

The recommended time frames for these follow-up visits are as follows:

- **Years 1 and 2:** Every 3 to 6 months
- **Years 3, 4, and 5:** Every 6 to 12 months
- **After year 5:** Once a year or as agreed upon with your provider

Time frame ranges are used to allow for differences in individual risk of recurrence and in patient and provider preference. Those considered at higher risk of recurrence may benefit from more frequent exams than those with a lower risk.

After the fifth year, visits are generally spaced out to once per year. Or you and your doctor may agree on a different schedule after discussing your personal risk of recurrence.

Imaging

Imaging generally isn't needed at regular intervals for an extended time after treatment. It is typically ordered if you have new or worsening symptoms, or if other findings suggest recurrence or spread. Follow-up imaging is described below according to the cancer stage.

Stage 1

If you had radiation or chemoradiation after non–fertility-sparing treatment, or if the cancer is stage 1B3, you may have a fluorodeoxyglucose (FDG) positron emission tomography/computed tomography (FDG-PET/CT) scan 3 to 6 months after finishing treatment. The area from the neck to the midthigh is typically scanned.

After fertility-sparing treatment, you may have an MRI of your pelvis (with contrast) 6 months after surgery and then yearly for 2 to 3 years.

Stages 2, 3, and 4A

Imaging is recommended 3 to 6 months after treatment for stage 2, 3, and 4A cervical cancers. An FDG-PET/CT scan is preferred, but a CT with contrast is also a recommended option. The area from the neck to the mid-thigh will be scanned.

Other imaging for these stages may include a pelvic MRI (with and without contrast) 3 to 6 months after finishing treatment.

Metastatic cancer

For stage 4B or distant recurrences of cervical cancer, imaging is used mainly to learn how the cancer is responding to systemic therapy. Imaging may include CT, MRI, or PET/CT.

Pap tests

Depending on the type of surgery you have (if any), you may have annual Pap screening tests after treatment. Pap testing is helpful for finding new areas of abnormal and precancerous cells. It isn't as good at detecting recurrent cervical cancer. Pap testing is also known as cervical or vaginal cytology.

Blood tests

If you develop symptoms, or if a physical exam is suspicious for recurrence, your provider may order blood tests.

In addition to a complete blood count (CBC), testing may measure blood urea nitrogen (BUN) and creatinine levels. These check your kidney function. Liver function tests may also be ordered.

Survivorship

In addition to surveillance testing, a range of other care is important for cancer survivors. This includes keeping alert for symptoms of cancer recurrence. For more information, see the chapter of this resource about survivorship.

We want your feedback!

Our goal is to provide helpful and easy-to-understand information on cancer. Take our survey to let us know what we got right and what we could do better.
NCCN.org/patients/feedback

Recurrence

This section discusses cervical cancer that doesn't improve with treatment (persistent) or that returns after treatment (recurrent). If your provider suspects recurrence based on your symptoms or a physical exam, you will have imaging tests to check.

If needed, exploratory surgery can help guide care decisions. This is surgery to look inside the body and learn the extent of the cancer.

Biomarker testing

Biomarkers are features of a cancer that can help guide treatment. Many are mutations (changes) in particular genes.

Biomarker testing is recommended for all recurrent cervical cancers. The results can be used to determine whether you can join certain clinical trials, and whether you may benefit from specific targeted therapies.

Some providers order biomarker testing early in the course of treatment. Others wait and order it only if the cancer returns or spreads.

When possible, testing should be performed on tumor tissue removed during a biopsy or surgery. Otherwise, a sample of blood may be tested instead.

Testing for PD-L1 expression is recommended for everyone with recurrent, progressive, or metastatic cervical cancer. If the PD-L1 level exceeds a set cutoff point, the cancer is considered PD-L1-positive.

The biomarkers listed below are less common in cervical cancer but should still be tested for.

- HER2
- Mismatch repair (MMR)
- Microsatellite instability (MSI)
- Tumor mutational burden (TMB)
- *NTRK* gene fusion (for those with a cervical sarcoma)
- *RET* gene fusion

If cancer returns to the pelvis

Cervical cancer that returns to the pelvis only is known as a local or regional recurrence. If the area hasn't been treated with radiation and the cancer can be surgically removed, this is generally preferred. After surgery, EBRT and systemic therapy are recommended. Brachytherapy may also be given.

If the area has already been treated with radiation and it is no longer an option, possible treatment options are listed below. The best option(s) for you will depend on the specific location of the new cancer growth in the pelvis.

- Pelvic exenteration surgery
- Radical hysterectomy
- Brachytherapy
- Individualized EBRT and possibly systemic therapy
- Systemic therapy
- Resection of new cancer growth

Radical hysterectomy and brachytherapy are typically only considered in carefully selected patients. Supportive care is always an option, whether you are in active treatment or not.

Pelvic exenteration

Pelvic exenteration is a radical surgery that involves removing all remaining organs of the reproductive system. This includes the uterus, fallopian tubes, ovaries, and vagina. Nearby organs including the bladder, rectum, and anus may also be removed. The goal is to cure the cancer by removing all the organs to which cancer has or may spread.

Vaginal reconstruction

It's often possible to reconstruct the vagina after pelvic exenteration. A surgeon can create an artificial vagina using muscle from another area of your body, often a muscle in the lower abdomen called the rectus abdominus. This procedure is sometimes referred to as muscle flap reconstruction.

If the bladder is removed

If the bladder or organs involved in bowel function are removed, a diversion is typically performed. Diversions are surgical procedures that divert (redirect) urine and stool to new openings through which they exit the body.

In an ileal (incontinent) conduit, after the bladder is removed, your surgeon will create a new tube from a piece of intestine (ileum). This tube will allow your kidneys to drain. Your urine will now exit the body through a small opening called a stoma. A small disposable bag attached to the outside of your abdomen collects the urine. This is called an ostomy bag or ostomy pouch. The bag stays attached to your body with the help of an adhesive part called a "wafer." The wafer sticks to the skin and acts as a watertight barrier.

Another way urine may be redirected after removing the bladder is a continent urinary diversion. Also called an artificial bladder or "Indiana pouch," this method uses a segment of intestine to create a pouch to hold urine. The pouch has a channel for urine to pass through that connects it to the wall of the abdomen.

A stoma is made in the abdominal wall at the location of the reservoir. Sometimes it can be made in the belly button, making it less noticeable. To drain urine, a catheter is inserted into the reservoir several times a day. A benefit of an artificial bladder is that you don't need an ostomy bag.

If the rectum is removed

If the rectum is removed, a permanent colostomy may be created. A colostomy connects the remaining colon to the outside of the abdomen. Stool exits the body through a stoma and goes into a bag attached to the skin.

In some cases, the remaining colon can be connected to the remaining rectum or anus. In this case a permanent colostomy may not be required and you may retain near-normal bowel function. But if the anus is removed, a permanent colostomy is always needed.

If both the bowel and bladder are removed

If both urinary and fecal diversion are needed, a double-barreled wet colostomy (DBWC) is sometimes used. In this technique, urine and stool are kept separate until they exit the body through the same stoma (opening). This method may have fewer leaks compared to having separate urinary and fecal diversions.

Metastatic cancer

Cervical cancer that isn't diagnosed early enough, or that is left untreated, often spreads to the liver, lungs, or bones. If this occurs, the cancer is described as metastatic.

If the cancer had already metastasized when it was found, it is stage 4B. If the cancer returns and metastasizes after treatment, it is called a distant recurrence. The information in this section applies to both.

Systemic therapy helps limit tumor growth and prevent further spread. Choosing the best systemic therapy for you begins with biomarker testing (if not already performed). Whether the cancer has the PD-L1 biomarker plays a key role in selecting a first-line regimen. **See Guide 1.**

If you can't have any of the preferred regimens, there are other recommended first-line regimens.

Local therapies

Local therapies are often an option for treating or controlling metastatic cancer, alone or with systemic therapy. These methods remove or destroy new cancer growth where it forms. Resection (surgery), external radiation therapy, and ablative therapies are types of local therapies.

Ablative therapies destroy areas of cancer with little harm to nearby tissue. They are often delivered using a probe or electrode placed directly into or next to the tumor.

Stereotactic body radiation therapy (SBRT) is a highly specialized type of radiation therapy that may be used to treat tumors in the liver, lungs, or bone. Only a few treatment sessions are needed.

Guide 1
Preferred* first-line regimens for recurrent or metastatic cervical cancer

Preferred for PD-L1-positive tumors	Pembrolizumab (Keytruda) + cisplatin (or carboplatin) + paclitaxel This regimen may also include bevacizumab, a biologic therapy designed to work with chemotherapy
Preferred for other tumor types	• Cisplatin (or carboplatin) + paclitaxel + bevacizumab • Atezolizumab (Tecentriq) + cisplatin (or carboplatin) + paclitaxel + bevacizumab

*Preferred regimens have been found to work better than other recommended regimens. They may also be safer.

Second-line or beyond

If first-line therapy doesn't work well, or stops working, you can switch to a second-line regimen. At this time, there are 2 preferred options:

- Tisotumab vedotin-tftb (Tivdak)
- Pembrolizumab (only preferred for cancers that are TMB-H, PD-L1-positive, or MSI-H/dMMR)

For cancers with a different biomarker, immunotherapy or targeted therapy may be an option. Biomarkers and their related systemic therapies are listed in **Guide 2.**

You may also consider enrolling in a clinical trial. Ask your treatment team if there is an open clinical trial that you can join.

If immunotherapy is planned, see the *NCCN Guidelines for Patients for Immunotherapy Side Effects: Immune Checkpoint Inhibitors* at NCCN.org/patientguidelines and on the NCCN Patient Guides for Cancer app.

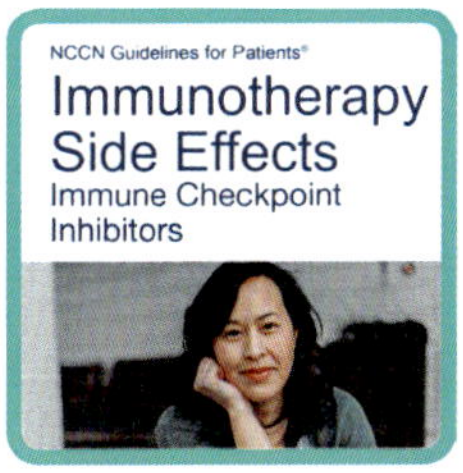

Guide 2
Biomarkers and their related treatments

Biomarker	Targeted therapy options
PD-L1 positive	• Nivolumab (Opdivo) • Tisotumab vedotin-tftv (Tivdak) + pembrolizumab (Keytruda)
HER2-positive	Fam-trastuzumab deruxtecan-nxki (Enhertu)
HER2-mutant	Neratinib (Nerlynx)
***RET* gene fusion-positive**	Selpercatinib (Retevmo)
***NTRK* gene fusion-positive**	• Larotrectinib (Vitrakvi) • Entrectinib (Rozlytrek) • Repotrectinib (Augtyro)

Supportive care

Supportive care is available to everyone with metastatic cervical cancer, regardless of whether you are in active treatment. Supportive care refers to a range of care and resources often needed by those with metastatic cancer. Hospice care, access to pain specialists, and emotional and spiritual support are all components of supportive care.

Because metastatic cancer cannot be cured, the main goal of supportive care is to make you more comfortable and to help keep the cancer under control. Supportive care may also help you live longer and feel better overall. When used for advanced cancers, supportive care is often called palliative care.

Advance care planning

Talking with your doctor about your prognosis can help with treatment planning. If the cancer cannot be controlled or cured, a care plan for the end of life can be made. Benefits of advance care planning include:

- Knowing what to expect
- Making the most of your time
- Lowering the stress of caregivers
- Having your wishes followed
- Having a better quality of life

Advance care planning starts with an honest talk between you and your doctors. Just having a general idea of your prognosis will help you decide at what point you may want to stop treatment, if at all.

Key points

- Treatment for early-stage cervical cancer often involves hysterectomy. External beam radiation therapy (EBRT) or chemoradiation may follow surgery. If you can't have surgery, EBRT and brachytherapy are recommended.
- Fertility-sparing treatment may be an option for some stage 1 cancers. Treatment typically involves either cone biopsy or radical trachelectomy.
- Extra imaging or surgical staging may be done for locally advanced cancers to see if there is cancer in lymph nodes. Treatment with chemoradiation and brachytherapy is recommended for most locally advanced cervical cancers.
- Surveillance after treatment involves physical exams and staying alert for symptoms of recurrence or spread.
- Follow-up imaging is recommended 3 to 6 months after finishing treatment for stage 2, 3, or 4A cancer. After that, imaging will be ordered if you have symptoms or there are other possible signs of relapse.
- If you haven't had treatment with EBRT, it is often used to treat cancer that returns to the pelvis. If the cancer can't be treated with radiation, pelvic exenteration surgery may be an option.
- For metastatic cancer, systemic therapy helps limit tumor growth and prevent further spread. Biomarker testing is used to help choose the best regimen(s) for you. Local therapies may be used to remove or destroy new cancer growth.

Questions to ask

- If surgery is planned, am I a candidate for fertility-sparing treatment?
- What symptoms should I look out for during treatment?
- How likely is it that the cancer will return?
- Has my tumor been sent for biomarker testing? Does the cancer have any biomarkers?

6

Treatment for neuroendocrine carcinoma of the cervix

This chapter describes the treatment options for a rare type of cervical cancer called neuroendocrine carcinoma of the cervix (NECC). Treatment often involves chemotherapy, external radiation therapy, and brachytherapy. Surgery may be an option for small cancers.

The most common type, small cell NECC, is the focus of this chapter. Treatment often involves chemotherapy, alone or as part of chemoradiation. The following regimens are preferred for chemotherapy:

- cisplatin and etoposide
- carboplatin and etoposide

If you can't have either of these, there are other recommended options. For chemoradiation, cisplatin and etoposide is preferred. If you can't have cisplatin, carboplatin is often used instead.

NECC tumors can contain cells from more common types of cervical cancer, including squamous cell carcinoma. In this case, the cancer is treated as NECC.

Enrolling in a clinical trial allows you to receive treatment while helping researchers learn more about this rare cancer. Ask your care team if you qualify for any current clinical trials. For more information, see the end of *Chapter 4: Types of treatment*.

Early NECC

NECC that hasn't spread beyond the cervix is stage 1. Treatment is guided by the size of the tumor.

Tumors 4 cm or smaller

Stage 1A1 and 1B2 cancers are 4 cm or smaller. If you are able to have surgery, radical hysterectomy is recommended. Nearby lymph nodes in the pelvis, and sometimes in the abdomen, will be removed for testing.

After surgery, treatment with either chemotherapy or chemoradiation is recommended.

A second option for tumors 4 cm or smaller is treatment with chemoradiation and brachytherapy. When treatment is over, your provider may recommend more chemotherapy.

Tumors larger than 4 cm

Tumors in the cervix that are larger than 4 cm are stage 1B3. The preferred treatment plan for these tumors begins with chemoradiation and brachytherapy. More chemotherapy may follow.

Another possibility is that chemotherapy will be given first to try to shrink the cancer. If chemotherapy works well, radical hysterectomy may be your next treatment. If you have this surgery, treatment with EBRT alone or chemoradiation may be given next. More chemotherapy may follow.

If radical hysterectomy isn't performed, treatment with chemoradiation and brachytherapy is the next step. More chemotherapy may follow.

Locally advanced NECC

The term locally advanced is used to describe cervical cancer that has grown beyond the uterus but hasn't spread to the liver, lungs, or bone. Stage 2, 3, and 4A NECC are locally advanced. These cancers are non-metastatic.

At this time, treatment with chemoradiation and brachytherapy is preferred for locally advanced NECC. When these treatments are over, you may have more chemotherapy with the same regimen.

The other recommended treatment strategy for locally advanced NECC is having chemotherapy first, followed by chemoradiation and brachytherapy.

If initial treatment works well, surveillance will begin. Surveillance involves testing to look for early signs of recurrence. The surveillance strategy for more common types of cervical cancer is also recommended for NECC.

Persistent cancer

If the cancer doesn't improve with initial treatment, it is described as persistent.

Persistent NECC is typically treated with systemic therapy. Pelvic exenteration surgery may also be an option to discuss with your provider. This radical surgery involves removing multiple organs from the pelvis. The goal is to cure the cancer by removing all of the organs to which cancer has or may spread.

Supportive care is also an option and is available to everyone with cancer. This care refers to a range of resources, such as hospice care, access to pain specialists, and emotional and spiritual support.

Standard of care is the best-known way to treat a particular disease based on past clinical trials. There may be more than one treatment regimen that is considered standard of care. Ask your care team what treatment options are available and if a clinical trial might be right for you.

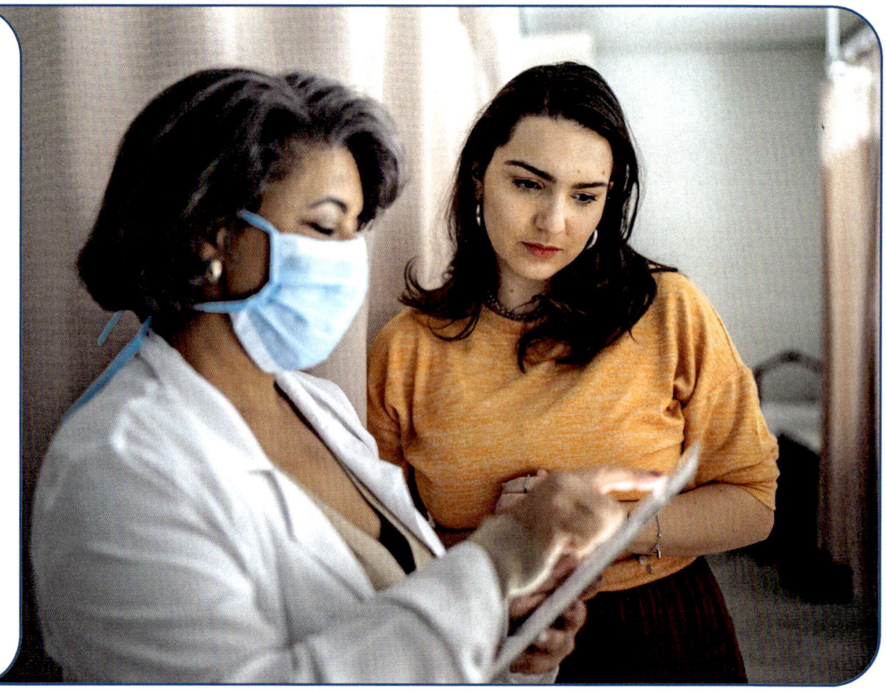

Recurrence or spread

If the cancer returns to the same area after treatment, systemic therapy and pelvic exenteration surgery are often options.

If the cancer spreads to the liver, lungs, or bone (metastasizes), systemic therapy is recommended to keep the cancer under control and prevent further spread. Recommended first-line regimens are listed in **Guide 3.**

Guide 3
First-line regimens for recurrent or metastatic small cell NECC

Preferred* regimens	• Cisplatin and etoposide • Carboplatin and etoposide
Other recommended regimens	• Cisplatin + etoposide + atezolizumab (Tecentriq) or durvalumab (Imfinzi) • Carboplatin + etoposide + atezolizumab or durvalumab • Topotecan + paclitaxel + bevacizumab • Cisplatin and paclitaxel • Carboplatin and paclitaxel (an option if you've received prior cisplatin therapy)

*Preferred regimens have been found to work better than other recommended regimens. They may also be safer.

Key points

- Small cell neuroendocrine carcinoma of the cervix (NECC) is a rare and usually fast-growing type of cervical cancer.
- Treatment for NECC often involves chemotherapy, external beam radiation therapy (EBRT), and brachytherapy. Surgery (along with other treatment) may also be an option for stage 1 NECC.
- Options for treating persistent or recurrent NECC that is only in the pelvis include systemic therapy and possibly pelvic exenteration surgery.
- Supportive care is an option for everyone with NECC. Talk to your care team about resources available to you.
- There is much to be learned about rare cancers like small cell NECC. Think about enrolling in a clinical trial for treatment.

Questions to ask

- Am I a candidate for surgery?
- Do you know of any available clinical trials I am eligible for?
- What are the side effects of the preferred systemic therapy regimens?

7 Survivorship

Survivorship focuses on the physical, emotional, and financial issues unique to cancer survivors. Survivorship begins at diagnosis and continues through treatment, recurrence, and end of life.

During and after cancer treatment, your primary care provider and your oncologist will work together to make sure you receive recommended care. But, you also have a responsibility—paying close attention to your body.

Staying alert for recurrence or spread

If cervical cancer does come back, it may affect your body in ways that you can feel or notice (symptoms). Your provider will teach you about the symptoms that may mean cervical cancer has returned or spread. They include:

- Vaginal discharge or bleeding
- Blood in your urine or stool
- Loss of appetite or weight loss
- Pain in the pelvis, hips, back, or legs
- Coughing
- Shortness of breath
- Swelling in your stomach or legs

If you notice any of these symptoms, contact your doctor right away. Do not wait for your next scheduled visit.

Late and long-term effects

Some side effects of cervical cancer treatment can start early and linger longer than expected. Others may not appear until long after treatment is over.

Many cervical cancer survivors experience changes in bowel, urinary, and sexual function. More general effects such as fatigue, trouble breathing, and difficulty sleeping (insomnia) are also common. The extent and degree of symptoms vary widely between patients. Ask your treatment team for a complete list of possible late and long-term side effects.

Bowel and bladder changes

Urinary incontinence (the inability to hold urine in the bladder) and urgency (a sudden, strong need to urinate) are possible after surgery or radiation therapy for cervical cancer. Watery and/or frequent bowel movements (diarrhea) are also possible.

Occasional bleeding may occur either with urination or bowel movements. Pelvic floor physical therapy, described next, can help with bowel and bladder changes.

Ostomy care

If you have an ostomy, you may want to join an ostomy support group. Another option is to see a health care provider who specializes in ostomy care, such as an ostomy nurse. People with ostomies can still live very active lifestyles. Consider consulting with an ostomy professional before undertaking vigorous physical activity.

Pelvic floor physical therapy

The pelvic floor is a group of muscles that supports the organs of the pelvis. These muscles play a key role in bowel and bladder control as well as sexual function and arousal.

There are ways to strengthen these muscles before and after treatment. This is known as pelvic floor physical therapy, and there are health care professionals who specialize in it. Pelvic floor therapy can include at-home exercises to tighten and release the vaginal and anal muscles (Kegel exercises) as well as hands-on techniques by a physical therapist.

Ask your care team for help finding a pelvic floor specialist in your area.

Infertility and early menopause

In premenopausal people, surgically removing the ovaries or exposing them to radiation causes a sudden drop in estrogen and progesterone. This results in infertility, and possibly menopausal symptoms. Your periods may stop and you may experience hot flashes, night sweats, weight gain, and mood changes.

The lining of the vagina can become thin, dry, and inflamed. This is called vaginal atrophy. Not having enough estrogen can also have long-term risks, including heart disease and bone loss (osteoporosis).

Premature menopause

If you are premenopausal, surgically removing the ovaries or exposing them to radiation can cause symptoms of menopause, including sleeping problems. Consulting with a menopause specialist is recommended.

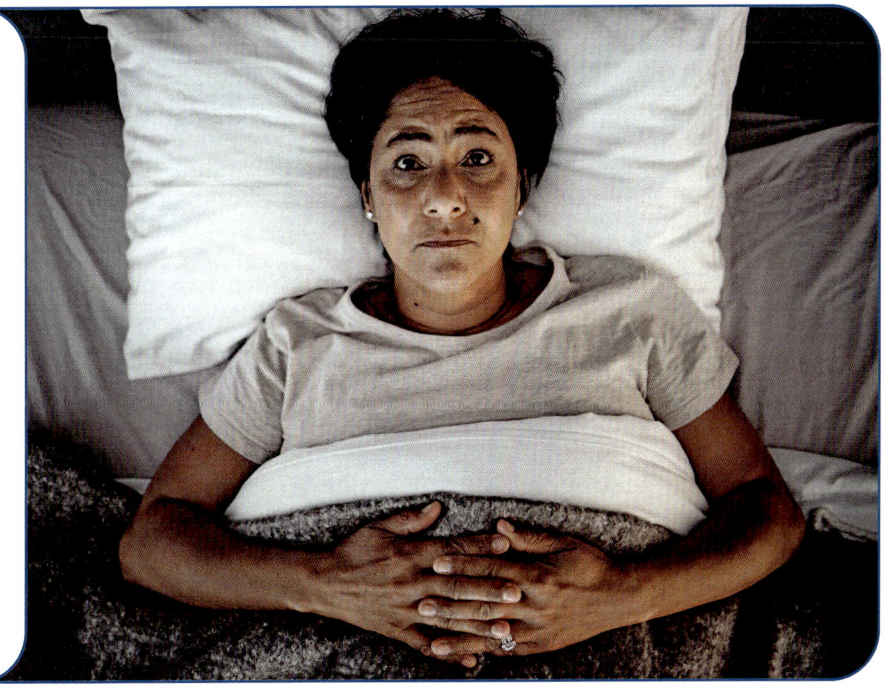

When these hormonal changes cause symptoms of menopause, menopausal hormone therapy (MHT) may be an option. This can include systemic (oral or intravenous) estrogen (combined with progestins for those with a uterus intact) and vaginal applications of estrogen. Speaking with a specialized menopausal symptom team may be helpful to determine whether MHT is right for you.

Vaginal moisturizers

Older age, menopause, and some cervical cancer treatments can cause the vagina to become dry and less stretchy. To offset this side effect, use of water-based vaginal moisturizers is highly encouraged.

Like moisturizers for your body, vaginal moisturizers restore moisture to the vagina and help to keep the vaginal tissue healthy. Vaginal moisturizers can be used daily. Many come with applicators to make using them easier. Vaginal estrogen cream or tablets may be particularly helpful where there has been thinning of the vaginal and vulvar tissues due to loss of estrogen.

Vaginal dilator therapy

Radiation therapy to the pelvis can cause the vagina to become shorter and narrower. This is called vaginal stenosis. Vaginal stenosis can make it uncomfortable or even painful to have sex, or to have vaginal exams by a doctor.

Using a vaginal dilator can prevent or treat vaginal stenosis. This is a device used to gradually stretch or widen the vagina. You can start using one as soon as 2 to 4 weeks after radiation therapy has ended, and continue to use it for as long as you want.

Sexual health

Sexual side effects can occur after cervical cancer treatment, including:

- Reduced sex drive (libido)
- Vaginal dryness
- Pain during sex
- Narrowing and shortening of the vagina (vaginal stenosis)

While it may be uncomfortable to talk about sexual health, keep in mind that these side effects are common and can often be managed or lessened. Consider seeing a sexual health therapist. These health care professionals specialize in helping cancer survivors and others overcome and manage sexual side effects of cancer treatment.

Many cancer treatment centers have programs focused solely on sexual health after cancer treatment. Ask your doctor about resources available through your cancer center that can help minimize the impact of cancer treatment on your sexual health.

Mental health and wellness

It can be hard to cope with the effects of cancer and its treatment. Many survivors report having a lower quality of life after cancer treatment. Depression, anxiety, fear of recurrence, and trouble adjusting to changes in the body are possible. Many people also have financial stressors, such as concerns or hesitation about returning to work and insurance coverage issues. Personal relationships, sexuality, and intimacy may also be affected by a cancer diagnosis or cancer treatment.

If you are anxious, distressed, depressed, or are just having trouble coping with life after cancer, you are not alone. Expect your treatment team to ask about your mental health. If they don't, speak up. There are resources available that can improve mental health and wellness for cancer survivors. The social workers at your treatment center can often help.

Weakened bones

Radiation treatment to the pelvis can weaken bones in the pelvis, putting you at increased risk of fractures. Your doctor may want to start monitoring the density of your bones.

Nerve damage

Chemotherapy can damage the sensory nerves. This is known as neuropathy. The damage can result in pain, numbness, tingling, swelling, or muscle weakness in different parts of the body. It often begins in the hands or feet and gets worse over time. Neuropathic pain is often described as a shooting or burning pain.

Swelling

Treatment for cervical cancer often involves removing lymph nodes during surgery. Lymph may not drain properly after lymph nodes are removed. This can result in lymphedema. Lymphedema is swelling caused by a build-up of lymph fluid in tissues. It most often occurs in the lower part of the body for cervical cancer survivors.

Healthy habits

Monitoring for the return of cervical cancer is important after finishing treatment. But it is also important to keep up with other aspects of your health. Steps you can take to help prevent other health issues and to improve your quality of life are described next.

Get screened for other types of cancer, such as breast, skin, and colorectal cancer. Talk to your primary care provider about recommended cancer screening tests for your age and risk level.

Get other recommended health care such as blood pressure screening and hepatitis C screening, and immunizations (such as the flu shot).

Leading a healthy lifestyle includes maintaining a healthy body weight. Exercising at a moderate intensity for at least 150 minutes per week is recommended. Talk to your doctor before starting a new exercise regimen. Try to eat a healthy diet that includes lots of plant-based foods.

Alcohol may increase the risk of certain cancers. Drink little to no alcohol.

If you use tobacco, quit! Your doctor can provide (or refer you for) counseling on how to stop smoking.

More information

For more information on cancer survivorship, the following NCCN Guidelines for Patients are available at NCCN.org/patientguidelines and on the NCCN Patient Guides for Cancer app.

- *Survivorship Care for Healthy Living*
- *Survivorship Care for Cancer-Related Late and Long-Term Effects*

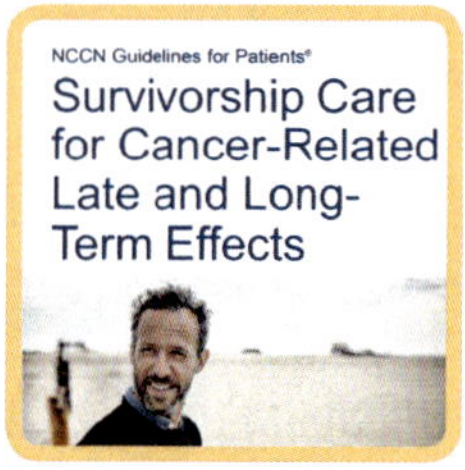

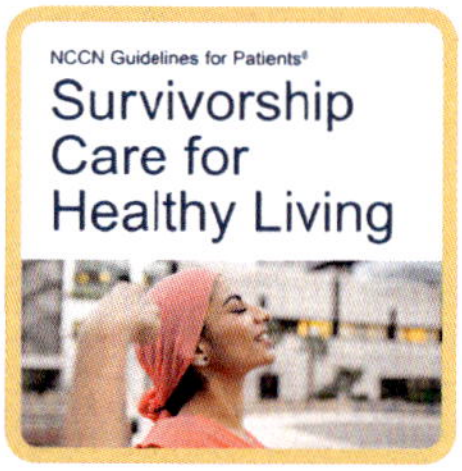

Key points

- Survivorship focuses on the physical, emotional, and financial issues unique to cancer survivors. Ask your cancer provider about a survivorship care plan. This plan helps your providers coordinate your follow-up care.
- It's important to stay alert for signs of potential recurrence or spread, including vaginal discharge or bleeding, blood in your urine or stool, and weight loss.
- Many survivors experience problems with bowel, urinary, and sexual function. Other physical side effects can include infertility, early menopause, fatigue, trouble breathing, insomnia, painful nerve damage, and swelling of the legs.
- Pelvic floor physical therapy, menopausal hormone therapy (MHT), and vaginal moisturizers and dilators can help with some side effects. Sexual health therapists help cancer survivors and others overcome and manage sexual side effects of cancer treatment.
- Depression, anxiety, fear of recurrence, and trouble adjusting to changes in the body are possible after cervical cancer treatment. Ask your care team about resources that can improve your mental health and wellness.

8
Other resources

Want to learn more? Here's how you can get additional help.

What else to know

This book can help you improve your cancer care. It plainly explains expert recommendations and suggests questions to ask your care team. But it's not the only resource that you have.

You're welcome to receive as much information and help as you need. Many people are interested in learning more about:

- The details of their health and treatment
- Being a part of a care team
- Getting financial help
- Finding a care provider who is an expert in their field
- Coping with health problems

What else to do

Your health care center can help you with next steps. They often have on-site resources to help meet your needs and find answers to your questions. Health care centers can also inform you of resources in your community.

In addition to help from your providers, the resources listed in the next section provide support for many people like yourself. Look through the list and visit the provided websites to learn more about these organizations.

Where to get help

Cancer*Care*
cancercare.org

Cancer Hope Network
cancerhopenetwork.org

Cervivor
cervivor.org

HPV Cancers Alliance
hpvalliance.org

Imerman Angels
imermanangels.org

National Coalition for Cancer Survivorship
canceradvocacy.org

Ovarian Cancer Research Alliance (OCRA)
ocrahope.org

Triage Cancer
triagecancer.org

Questions to ask

- Who can I talk to about help with housing, food, and other basic needs?
- What help is available for transportation, childcare, and home care?
- Are there other services available to me and my caregivers?

Words to know

abdomen
The belly area between the chest and pelvis.

adenocarcinoma
Cervical cancer that starts in glandular cells in the endocervix. About 1 in 5 cervical cancers is an adenocarcinoma.

adenosquamous carcinoma
A less common type of cervical cancer that contains both squamous cells and gland-like cells.

biomarker
Features of a cancer that can help guide your treatment. Many biomarkers are mutations (changes) in the DNA of cancer cells.

brachytherapy
A type of radiation therapy in which radioactive material sealed in needles, seeds, wires, or catheters is placed directly into or near a tumor. Also called internal radiation therapy.

cancer stage
A rating of the extent of cancer in the body.

cervical intraepithelial neoplasia (CIN)
Abnormal and potentially pre-cancerous cells on the surface of the cervix. Also called cervical dysplasia.

cervix
The lower part of the uterus that connects to the vagina.

clinical trial
Research on an investigational test or treatment to assess its safety or how well it works.

cone biopsy
A procedure in which a cone-shaped piece of abnormal tissue is removed from the cervix. May be used to gather more information about the extent of a cancer or to treat some early cervical cancers. Also called cervical conization.

ectocervix
The rounded, outer part of the cervix that extends into the vagina. The ectocervix is lined with cells called squamous cells.

endocervix
The inner part of the cervix that forms a canal between the vagina and the uterus. The endocervix is lined with columnar (glandular) cells that make mucus.

external beam radiation therapy (EBRT)
Treatment with radiation received from a large machine outside the body. Types of EBRT include intensity-modulated radiation therapy (IMRT) and stereotactic body radiation therapy (SBRT).

gynecologic oncologist
A surgeon who is an expert in cancers that start in the female reproductive organs.

human papillomavirus (HPV)
A common sexually transmitted infection. Almost all cervical cancers are caused by long-term HPV infection.

induction chemotherapy
Chemotherapy given before planned treatment with chemoradiation.

intensity-modulated radiation therapy (IMRT)
An advanced type of external radiation therapy often used to treat cervical cancer. Allows a high dose of radiation to reach the tumor while limiting the amount that reaches surrounding normal tissue and nearby organs and structures.

lymph
A clear fluid containing white blood cells that fight infection and disease.

lymph nodes
Small groups of disease-fighting cells located throughout the body.

lymphovascular space invasion (LVSI)
The presence of tumor cells in the blood vessels or lymph vessels inside the tumor. LVSI is a risk factor for cancer spread.

medical oncologist
A doctor who is an expert in treating cancer with systemic therapies, such as chemotherapy.

metastasis
The spread of cancer cells from the first tumor to another body part.

neuroendocrine carcinoma of the cervix (NECC)
A rare and often fast-growing type of cervical cancer.

neuropathy
A nerve problem that causes pain, tingling, and numbness in the hands and feet.

ovarian transposition
Surgery that moves one or both ovaries out of the range of the radiation beam. Also called oophoropexy.

ovary
One of a pair of organs that make hormones and eggs for sexual reproduction.

parametrium
The fat and connective tissue surrounding the uterus. The parametrium helps connect the uterus to other tissues in the pelvis.

pathologist
An expert in testing cells and tissue to find disease.

pelvic exenteration
A radical surgery used to treat cervical cancer that returns to the pelvis. The uterus (including the cervix), vagina, ovaries, and fallopian tubes are removed. The bladder, rectum, and/or anus may also be removed.

pelvis
The area of the body between the hip bones.

platinum-based chemotherapy
Treatment with 2 or more chemotherapy drugs and the main drug is made with platinum.

premature menopause
The onset of menopause caused by removing the ovaries or exposing them to radiation. Results from the sudden drop in estrogen in the body.

radiation oncologist
A doctor who is an expert in treating cancer with radiotherapy.

radiologist
A doctor who is an expert in interpreting imaging tests.

recurrence
The return of cancer after treatment. Also called a relapse.

squamous cell carcinoma
Cancer that starts in squamous cells lining the ectocervix. The most common type of cervical cancer.

supportive care
A range of resources and care to improve quality of life for cancer survivors. Also called palliative care.

targeted therapy
Treatment with drugs that target a specific or unique feature of cancer cells.

trachelectomy
Surgery to remove the cervix. The upper part of the vagina and certain pelvic lymph nodes may also be removed.

transformation zone
The area where the endocervix and ectocervix meet. Most cervical cancers and pre-cancers start in the transformation zone. Also called the squamocolumnar junction.

Type A hysterectomy
Surgery to remove only the uterus (including the cervix). Most commonly used for very early cervical cancers. Also called simple hysterectomy.

Type B radical hysterectomy
Surgery to remove the uterus (including the cervix), some connective tissue that holds the cervix in place, and about a half inch or less of the vagina. Type B hysterectomy is performed through the abdomen. Also called modified radical hysterectomy.

Type C1 radical hysterectomy
Surgery to remove the uterus (including the cervix), much of the connective tissue that holds the cervix in place, and the top quarter or third of the vagina. Type C1 hysterectomy is performed through the abdomen.

uterus
The organ where a fetus grows and develops during pregnancy. Also called the womb.

NCCN Contributors

This patient guide is based on the NCCN Clinical Practice Guidelines in Oncology (NCCN Guidelines®) for Cervical Cancer, Version 4.2025. It was adapted, reviewed, and published with help from the following people:

Dorothy A. Shead, MS
Senior Director
Patient Information Operations

Erin Vidic, MA
Senior Medical Writer, Patient Information

Susan Kidney
Senior Graphic Design Specialist

The NCCN Clinical Practice Guidelines in Oncology (NCCN Guidelines®) for Cervical Cancer, Version 4.2025 were developed by the following NCCN Panel Members:

Nadeem R. Abu-Rustum, MD
Memorial Sloan Kettering Cancer Center

*Susana M. Campos, MD, MPH, MS
Dana-Farber/Brigham and Women's Cancer Center

*Sudha Amarnath, MD
Case Comprehensive Cancer Center/ University Hospitals Seidman Cancer Center and Cleveland Clinic Taussig Cancer Institute

Rebecca Arend, MD
O'Neal Comprehensive Cancer Center at UAB

Emma Barber, MD
Robert H. Lurie Comprehensive Cancer Center of Northwestern University

Kristin Bradley, MD
University of Wisconsin Carbone Cancer Center

Rebecca Brooks, MD
UC Davis Comprehensive Cancer Center

Junzo Chino, MD
Duke Cancer Institute

Hye Sook Chon, MD
Moffitt Cancer Center

Marta Ann Crispens, MD
Vanderbilt-Ingram Cancer Center

Shari Damast, MD
Yale Cancer Center/Smilow Cancer Hospital

Christine M. Fisher, MD, MPH
University of Colorado Cancer Center

*Peter Frederick, MD
Roswell Park Comprehensive Cancer Center

David K. Gaffney, MD, PhD
Huntsman Cancer Institute at the University of Utah

*Stephanie Gaillard, MD, PhD
Johns Hopkins Kimmel Cancer Center

Robert Giuntoli II, MD
Abramson Cancer Center at the University of Pennsylvania

*Scott Glaser, MD
City of Hope National Medical Center

Brooke E. Howitt, MD
Stanford Cancer Institute

Kari Kendra, MD, PhD/Liaison
The Ohio State University Comprehensive Cancer Center - James Cancer Hospital and Solove Research Institute

*Lisa Landrum, MD PhD
Indiana University Melvin and Bren Simon Comprehensive Cancer Center

Jayanthi Lea, MD
UT Southwestern Simmons Comprehensive Cancer Center

Nita Lee, MD, MPH
The UChicago Medicine Comprehensive Cancer Center

Gina Mantia-Smaldone, MD
Fox Chase Cancer Center

Andrea Mariani, MD
Mayo Clinic Comprehensive Cancer Center

David Mutch, MD
Siteman Cancer Center at Barnes-Jewish Hospital and Washington University School of Medicine

Christa Nagel, MD
The Ohio State University Comprehensive Cancer Center - James Cancer Hospital and Solove Research Institute

Larissa Nekhlyudov, MD, MPH
Dana-Farber/Brigham and Women's Cancer Center

Karina Nieto, MD
Case Comprehensive Cancer Center/ University Hospitals Seidman Cancer Center and Cleveland Clinic Taussig Cancer Institute

Chika Nwachukwu, MD, PhD
UC San Diego Moores Cancer Center

Mirna Podoll, MD
Vanderbilt-Ingram Cancer Center

Kerry Rodabaugh, MD
Fred & Pamela Buffett Cancer Center

Ritu Salani, MD, MBA
UCLA Jonsson Comprehensive Cancer Center

John Schorge, MD
St. Jude Children's Research Hospital/ The University of Tennessee Health Science Center

Scott Schuetze, MD, PhD
University of Michigan Rogel Cancer Center

Jean Siedel, DO, MS
University of Michigan Rogel Cancer Center

Rachel Sisodia, MD
Mass General Cancer Center

Pamela Soliman, MD, MPH
The University of Texas MD Anderson Cancer Center

Stefanie Ueda, MD
UCSF Helen Diller Family Comprehensive Cancer Center

Renata Urban, MD
Fred Hutchinson Cancer Center

*Emily Wyse
Patient Advocate

NCCN

Nicole McMillian, MS
Senior Guidelines Coordinator

Vaishnavi Sambandam, PhD
Oncology Scientist/Medical Writer

* Reviewed this patient guide.
For disclosures, visit NCCN.org/disclosures.

NCCN Cancer Centers

Abramson Cancer Center
at the University of Pennsylvania
Philadelphia, Pennsylvania
800.789.7366 • pennmedicine.org/cancer

Case Comprehensive Cancer Center/
University Hospitals Seidman Cancer Center and
Cleveland Clinic Taussig Cancer Institute
Cleveland, Ohio
UH Seidman Cancer Center
800.641.2422 • uhhospitals.org/services/cancer-services
CC Taussig Cancer Institute
866.223.8100 • my.clevelandclinic.org/departments/cancer
Case CCC
216.844.8797 • case.edu/cancer

City of Hope National Medical Center
Duarte, California
800.826.4673 • cityofhope.org

Dana-Farber/Brigham and Women's Cancer Center |
Mass General Cancer Center
Boston, Massachusetts
877.442.3324 • youhaveus.org
617.726.5130 • massgeneral.org/cancer-center

Duke Cancer Institute
Durham, North Carolina
888.275.3853 • dukecancerinstitute.org

Fox Chase Cancer Center
Philadelphia, Pennsylvania
888.369.2427 • foxchase.org

Fred & Pamela Buffett Cancer Center
Omaha, Nebraska
402.559.5600 • unmc.edu/cancercenter

Fred Hutchinson Cancer Center
Seattle, Washington
206.667.5000 • fredhutch.org

Huntsman Cancer Institute at the University of Utah
Salt Lake City, Utah
800.824.2073 • healthcare.utah.edu/huntsmancancerinstitute

Indiana University Melvin and Bren Simon
Comprehensive Cancer Center
Indianapolis, Indiana
888.600.4822 • www.cancer.iu.edu

Johns Hopkins Kimmel Cancer Center
Baltimore, Maryland
410.955.8964
www.hopkinskimmelcancercenter.org

Mayo Clinic Comprehensive Cancer Center
Phoenix/Scottsdale, Arizona
Jacksonville, Florida
Rochester, Minnesota
480.301.8000 • Arizona
904.953.0853 • Florida
507.538.3270 • Minnesota
mayoclinic.org/cancercenter

Memorial Sloan Kettering Cancer Center
New York, New York
800.525.2225 • mskcc.org

Moffitt Cancer Center
Tampa, Florida
888.663.3488 • moffitt.org

O'Neal Comprehensive Cancer Center at UAB
Birmingham, Alabama
800.822.0933 • uab.edu/onealcancercenter

Robert H. Lurie Comprehensive Cancer Center
of Northwestern University
Chicago, Illinois
866.587.4322 • cancer.northwestern.edu

Roswell Park Comprehensive Cancer Center
Buffalo, New York
877.275.7724 • roswellpark.org

Siteman Cancer Center at Barnes-Jewish Hospital
and Washington University School of Medicine
St. Louis, Missouri
800.600.3606 • siteman.wustl.edu

St. Jude Children's Research Hospital/
The University of Tennessee Health Science Center
Memphis, Tennessee
866.278.5833 • stjude.org
901.448.5500 • uthsc.edu

Stanford Cancer Institute
Stanford, California
877.668.7535 • cancer.stanford.edu

The Ohio State University Comprehensive Cancer Center -
James Cancer Hospital and Solove Research Institute
Columbus, Ohio
800.293.5066 • cancer.osu.edu

The UChicago Medicine Comprehensive Cancer Center
Chicago, Illinois
773.702.1000 • uchicagomedicine.org/cancer

The University of Texas MD Anderson Cancer Center
Houston, Texas
844.269.5922 • mdanderson.org

UC Davis Comprehensive Cancer Center
Sacramento, California
916.734.5959 • 800.770.9261
health.ucdavis.edu/cancer

UC San Diego Moores Cancer Center
La Jolla, California
858.822.6100 • cancer.ucsd.edu

UCLA Jonsson Comprehensive Cancer Center
Los Angeles, California
310.825.5268 • uclahealth.org/cancer

UCSF Helen Diller Family
Comprehensive Cancer Center
San Francisco, California
800.689.8273 • cancer.ucsf.edu

University of Colorado Cancer Center
Aurora, Colorado
720.848.0300 • coloradocancercenter.org

University of Michigan Rogel Cancer Center
Ann Arbor, Michigan
800.865.1125 • rogelcancercenter.org

University of Wisconsin Carbone Cancer Center
Madison, Wisconsin
608.265.1700 • uwhealth.org/cancer

UT Southwestern Simmons
Comprehensive Cancer Center
Dallas, Texas
214.648.3111 • utsouthwestern.edu/simmons

Vanderbilt-Ingram Cancer Center
Nashville, Tennessee
877.936.8422 • vicc.org

Yale Cancer Center/Smilow Cancer Hospital
New Haven, Connecticut
855.4.SMILOW • yalecancercenter.org

share with us.

Take our survey and help make the NCCN Guidelines for Patients better for everyone!

NCCN.org/patients/comments

Index

Made in United States
North Haven, CT
03 October 2025

80380759R00042